TO THE MARROW

TO THE MARROW

BY

ROBERT SEDER

CavanKerry Press LTD.

Library of Congress Cataloging-in-Publication Data

Seder, Robert, 1949-2002

To the marrow / by Robert Seder.-- 1st ed.

p. cm.

ISBN-13: 978-0-9723045-6-6

ISBN-10: 0-9723045-6-8

1. Seder, Robert, 1949-2002--Health. 2. Lymphoma--Patients--New York (State)--New York--Biography. 3. Bone marrow--Transplantation--New York (State)--New York--Patients--Care--Biography. I. Title.

RC280.L9.S43 2005

362.196'994410092--dc22

2005028139

Cover Art by Peter Cusack *To the Marrow* © 2005

Cover and book design by Peter Cusack

Author Photograph by Jean Churchill

First Edition

Printed in the United States of America

CavanKerry Press Ltd.

Fort Lee, New Jersey

www.cavankerrypress.org

LaurelBooks

To the Marrow is the third title of CavanKerry's Literature of Illness imprint. LaurelBooks are fine collections of poetry and prose that explore the many poignant issues associated with confronting serious physical and/or psychological illness.

CavanKerry is grateful to the Arnold P. Gold Foundation for the Advancement of Humanism in Medicine for joining us in sponsoring this imprint. Offering LaurelBooks as teaching tools to medical schools is the result of shared concerns—humanism, community, and meeting the needs of the underserved. Together with the Gold Foundation, CavanKerry's two outreach efforts, GiftBooks and Presenting Poetry & Prose, bring complimentary books and readings to the medical community at major hospitals across the United States.

The Arnold P. Gold Foundation

Discover JERSEY ARTS

NEW JERSEY STATE COUNCIL ON THE ARTS

CavanKerry Press is grateful for the support it receives from the New Jersey State Council on the Arts.

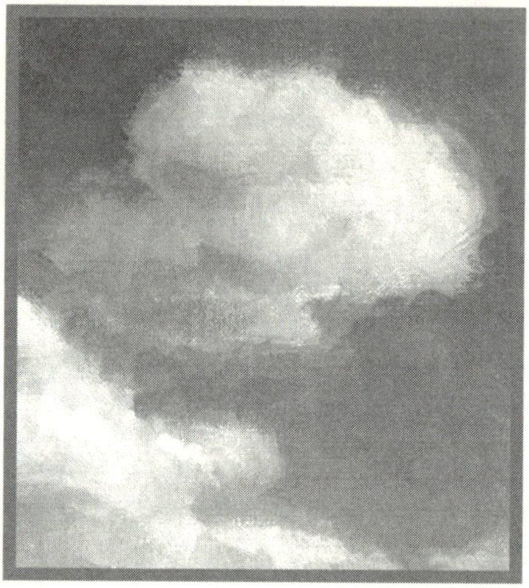

Acknowledgements

I am immensely grateful for the spectacular medical care I have obtained at Sloan-Kettering Memorial Hospital and Dana-Farber Cancer Institute of Boston during all the years of fighting cancer. I extend heartfelt thanks here to Doctors Lini Pandite, Rob Soiffer, Diane Stover and Gail Schattner; my good friend and neighbor Dr. Gerry Hurwitz; to Dr. Ted Alyea and Dr. Richard Collens, for their wisdom; and to those many first-rate nurses who have cared for me (especially Eugenie, Sandy, Kathy and Larry). The advice and guidance of Judy Nenner and Dr. Bob Abramson are essential to my well-being, such as it is. I extend huge thanks to Dr. Richard Seder and Dr. Kenneth Offit. For extraordinary support with my effort to create memoir out of transplant, I am grateful to my friends Celia Bland, Joan Bailey, Dorothy Crane, Bernard Greenwald, Paul Schaefer, my cousins Henry and Judy Grunebaum, and my sister Judy Erez. I give all my love, and thanks beyond measure, to Jean, my wife and my best friend.

—Robert Seder
January, 2002

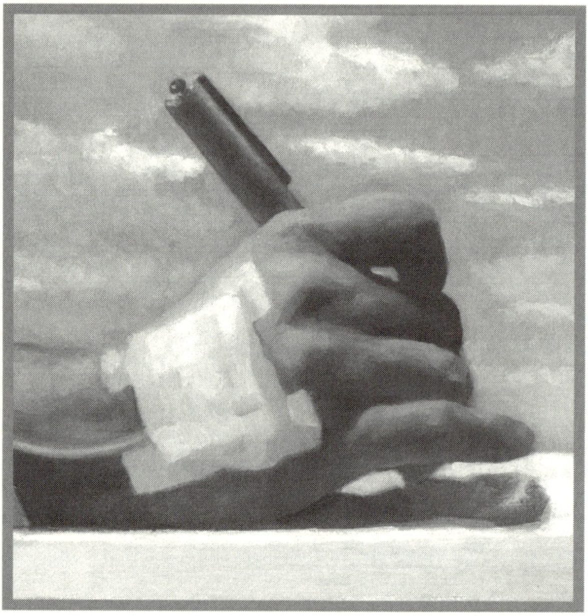

‡

Dedicated to the memory of my mother, Annette Ames Seder, who fought with her cancer, and won, for 28 years; and to my two children, Nathan and Clare, for whom I fight to the death to stay very much alive.

‡

This book is for all of the people facing cancer or a bone marrow transplant. I wish them all good luck and great strength in their battle to triumph over illness.

Table of Contents

Introduction by *Kenneth Offit M.D.* xiii
Foreword by *Mark Nepo* xvii
Day Minus Seven 3
Day Minus Six 7
Day Minus Five 11
Day Minus Four 14
Day Minus Three 18
Day Minus Two 22
Day Minus One 24
Day Zero 30
Day One 33
Day Two 39
Day Three 41
Day Four 50
Day Five 54
Day Six 57
Day Seven 60
Day Eight 63
Day Nine 68
Day Ten 70
Day Eleven 71
Day Twelve 74
Day Thirteen 77
Day Fourteen 80
Day Fifteen 87
Day Sixteen 91
Day Seventeen 92

Day Eighteen 96
Day Nineteen 99
Day Twenty 102
Day Twenty-one 108
Day Twenty-two 112
Day Twenty-three 114
Week Five 117
Week Six 121
Week Seven 125
Month Three 130
Month Four 136
Month Five 145
Month Six 148
Month Seven 152
Month Eight 156
Month Nine 159
Month Ten 161
Year Five 164

Afterward 172

Introduction

On the day of our graduation, every member of my class at the Harvard Medical School was handed a turn-of-the-century monograph by Dr. Frederick Cheever Shattuck. The old professor informed us that "no one gets as close to the real man as the doctor. The lawyer gets closer to his money . . . the clergyman . . . closer to the would-be than real self. The doctor sees plenty of evil, more weakness, but still more of good in human nature. While the head must rule the heart, the latter cannot go untouched."

My relationship with Robert Seder was intimately close but at the same time ruled by the head and not the heart. Chronicled in the pages that follow is a tale of one man's extraordinary grace, courage, and resounding epiphanies, set against the backdrop of the most complex and grueling medical interventions of the past century. This was the only time in my decades of medical practice that I treated a relative, albeit a distant one (my mother-in-law's second cousin). But from the start, my nurse Eugenie and I related to Robert Seder as if he were our closest kin. As Eugenie put it, he was special because he was one of those "people we just like because we like 'em." And this was true of every physician and nurse who reported back to me about Robert Seder.

As revealed in the saga that Bob Seder describes, it took a clear head as much as a good heart to navigate the complexities of bone marrow transplantation for lymphoma in the early 1990's. One of the top six most common cancers in the United States, the rate of lymphomas increased over 70% in the last two decades of the 20th century. This seemingly obscure cancer of the immune system claimed such notable victims as Jacqueline Kennedy Onassis and the Shah of Iran. While the most rapidly fatal types of lymphomas could be cured with intensive chemotherapy, the bitter irony then, and now, was that the so-called "indolent" lymphomas, which killed more slowly, could not be cured by traditional therapy. The story that follows marks an early attempt to change that grim fate by eradicating slow growing lymphomas with very high dose chemotherapy and total body irradiation, followed by a "rescue" of the patient with administration of portions of their own pre-collected marrow. Although peripheral stem cells from the blood instead of bone marrow are used today, and newer monoclonal antibody-based therapies are available, so-called autologous transplantation procedures are still widely administered in the treatment of relapsed lymphomas.

As Dr. Shattuck also warned his students: "Medicine is truly a science in that it rests upon the foundation of facts . . . It is true that the fact of today may not be a fact of tomorrow . . . the more we know the more we find we don't know." And so, at about the same time as Robert Seder was being treated at the Dana-Farber Cancer Center in Boston, another patient, and recent presidential candidate, was also being treated for the same disease. In 1992, just a year before Robert Seder's diagnosis with low-grade lymphoma, Senator Paul Tsongas said he was "cancer free" after a bone marrow transplant for low-grade lymphoma. There was a feeling of hope at that time that this disease had finally been toppled. While Robert Seder's own medical saga would ultimately follow a course remarkably similar to Senator Tsongas's, there was no way to know that "the best medicine of 1993," as Bob Seder put it, was still far from perfect.

However, the story that Robert Seder tells is one of a path and not an end. The meticulous attention to detail, emotional trials, and hidden epiphanies of the modern medical travail are rendered for us: the nausea meds, folic acid, needles, syringes, heparin, dressings, blood counts, Sunday Times, vomiting, transfusion, chemo, splash of sunlight on a bookshelf, birthday in an emergency room, the family always at his side, the kind social worker, the hug from the pregnant nurse, the intravenous antibiotics, fights with insurance companies over duplicate charges, a taste of basil and sundried tomatoes, and, finally, the view of sunlight hitting the tops of pine trees on a clear morning. I don't know if in Boston they still hand Dr. Shattuck's book to medical students on graduation day, but after you read Robert Seder's remarkable journey, you'll agree that this one would be a fine substitute.

—Kenneth Offit M.D.
Memorial Sloan-Kettering Hospital
August, 2005

Foreword

I cannot but say that my life, what's left of it,
is better for this new way of breathing . . .
—Robert Seder

To the Marrow is Robert Seder's intimate and searing journal of his five-year journey through a bone marrow transplant back into life, as if there is any going back. This book is heartbreaking in the best sense of the word. It will break your heart open and offer you the chance to not let your life evaporate around you or within you. The book is profound, not because Robert Seder has died, but because any time a human being opens the door between life and death and turns to let the light flood those coming behind, we see and hear things briefly with an echo of the gods who normally stay out of view. It is up to us whether we dismiss such illuminations or take them as the unseen bedrock of our days. In these pages, Robert Seder opens the most honest conversation with no one and everyone on what it means to be alive, and to love and be loved. In these pages, we witness how the ordinary days can press a heart like coal into the diamond that it is.

I didn't know Robert Seder, but I do now. As a cancer survivor myself, we would have had much to talk about. I also had lymphoma. I also had Cytoxan dripped into my veins. We had the same protocol of chemo, CHOP, and the same shot of Ativan to send us off. The poisons were welcomed because we were at the place where life and death are stitched and it's hard to know one from the other. I could have been in his bed after him. I'll never know why he had to go through this and I didn't. Or why his story has found me now. But as a cancer survivor, I couldn't help but rub my scars while reading of the blessed and difficult path he faced. Like a Holocaust survivor rubbing his tattoo each time he hears of another life tossed inside that storm, I kept leaning in to hear the hard-earned wisdom he was imparting till the end.

In the beginning of this journey, Robert cautions, "If one day you don't hear from me, don't assume the worst." The further we get from his death, the more this seems a philosophy of life. In a world where darkness and fear have become our daily bread, Robert Seder tells us, in the midst of terrible tunnels he was asked to shimmy through to stay here, that the best waits in what is unheard, in the quiet silence that holds us up. There is remarkable strength in listening past the worst; not skipping over it, but through it. This is one of the gifts this compassionate and clear man has given us.

As he enters hospitals and procedures, Robert is able to imagine the people who came before him, "nameless in (their) suffering." The forced isolation he faced (six weeks at the Dana-Farber Cancer Institute in Boston) provided him with a harsh, yet privileged ledge from which to view the world. Ironically, inside his solitary room he was given his own stethoscope and thermometer to monitor his heart and temperature. In deep ways, this book is the record of those readings, not just his own, but of the pulse of the living.

Once inside his isolated room, Robert declares, "I'm an elephant come home to die . . . Images of coming full circle look an awful lot like standing still." Elephants are regal, steadfast creatures, famous for their ability to keep moving while carrying the memory of their kind. In the Hindu tradition, they represent a deity, the provider and remover of obstacles, known as Ganesh. In this, Robert Seder named his role, almost with prescience. His daring to let us walk with him and suffer with him is a lesson in how to keep moving while preserving what is worth preserving, and how to move through and learn from the god of obstacles.

On the day he received his own marrow back into his bones, Robert wrote, "Myth has it that the marrow circulates through the bloodstream and finds its way back inside the bones where it belongs . . . I took a deep breath. Find your way home. Come back to me. I am home." This speaks to what we all face. For whatever the details of our dreams and their obstacles and whatever way life will rearrange us and transform us, the stuff that matters will find its way back inside our bones where it belongs, if we can stay true to what we know and what we love.

Along the way, we are in the room with him where life is but a flicker from flaring or going out. Along for the ride, we are privileged to witness his growing moments of tenderness and rawness, and the thinning of everything extraneous. In his isolation, he is not allowed to have even ice in his water, and, in the middle of the night, he misses "the comforting sound of the ice tinkling in the pitcher when they (would) wake me." Another day, his cousin Richard, a pathologist, comes to visit. "He apologizes for not staying longer, but (getting) eyeball to eyeball for a few minutes, that's what counts." After a tiresome visit, he accompanies his dear wife, Jean, in his mind, as she leaves and slouches in the hall. And when his father says little because there is little cheerful he can say, Robert writes, once he leaves, "But here's the thing, Dad, my knowing you are hurting might help me feel less alone . . . (It) doesn't have to be what I feel. But hurt lets me know I'm not alone. We are all holding it in. I am dying for a breath. A free, easy deep breath. A sigh, a shout." And when his longtime friend Denise comes, he is relieved. "We didn't say much, just held onto each other for nowhere long enough."

And so, as illness and crisis and the humble press of experience will do to even the most stubborn of us, Robert Seder found privacy to be an illusion. Only in not hiding what we feel do we find the strength to heal and go on, "I was long past the point of privacy, of—Don't talk about it and maybe it will go away."

It is a simple yet profound lesson that we seldom listen to, unless faced with death. "Life won't go away." The press of illness only makes the truth of this more acute. The only way out is through. And it is the passing through that holds the secret blessings, whether we die or live another day. In this, Robert Seder affirms that being human is the only way through. And being human not only bears but demands all the human moods—including fear, care, anger, peace, sadness, passion, detachment, and joy. It is our skin of humanness that lets us pass through such narrowing passages as this strange disease, cancer, in which we drink poisons to kill the disease and then strange brews to kill the poisons.

Yet, despite all he goes through, and, in some measure, because of all he goes through, Robert grows more alive inwardly, in the marrow, as his outer body weakens. His want to reach, and touch, and be touched, and share only grows stronger. "There is so much I want to tell you. The months of treatment. I have to tell you about my mother, and how I've lived with somebody's cancer most of my life. You'll want to know what I do when I'm not dealing with this, which I almost can't remember, and about my family, and what I'm reading. I want to tell you about the acupuncturist, the healer, and more about therapy. How am I going to get all this said?"

How do any of us get it all said? In the end, we don't say much, just hold onto each other for nowhere long enough. It is strange, but it happens from time to time. We meet a friend after they are gone. I count Robert Seder as such a friend who mirrored the enormous demands life can make on us, who showed in his honest account and tender resolve not to look away, that, hard as it is, we are well equipped to extract great meaning from what we are given.

Physically, the word marrow refers to the soft tissue that lives at the center of our bones. It is the source of our blood cells. Throughout the ages, the marrow, the soft source of blood within bone, has also served as a metaphor for the inmost, most life-giving part. It is the stuff that matters at the heart of what moves us through the world. In *To the Marrow*, Robert Seder shows us what matters and what carries it, and that what is soft and central not only survives, it is the only thing to survive when everything extraneous is worn away.

It is all any of us can hope for: to survive the wearing away and behold what is soft and central and lasting. Not free of struggle, but back in life, Robert admits, "I don't think that we who have been through this are heroes, and neither are the doctors, nurses, and caregivers saints. We are people hungry for life . . . (And) all you get for this enormous effort is more life. Life with all its shocks and heartaches . . . (But) the simple stuff of life is still here and still works . . . everything registers."

Like so many of life's great teachings, a moment opens from a scratch and widens to a cavern we might fall into, from which we are changed and rearranged until what is dark at the bottom becomes lighted. Not imagining he would serve this way, Robert Seder was such a guide. To journey with him will only make you softer and stronger.

—Mark Nepo
August, 2005

TO THE MARROW

DAY MINUS SEVEN

Tomorrow I walk into a room at the Dana-Farber Cancer Institute and will not walk out for four to six weeks. Every day I can, I'll let you know what happens as I undergo a bone marrow transplant. I understand there'll be some bad days when I won't feel like saying anything. If one day you don't hear from me, don't assume the worst. Maybe I'll just be too tired to talk.

While I'm in there, you will be out walking around in the world. Dress warmly for the January cold and wear your boots when you go out to eat and dance. Take care when you go to work, go on vacation, go shopping, go skating.

While I'm inside, you may get fired or start a new job, retire, graduate, or start school. You might go broke or win the lottery, get married or separated or come out of the closet.

You'll get sick, call the doctor, put off calling the doctor, get well. You'll fight with your family, make up, break up, crack up. You'll fall in love, keep old loves alive, watch love fade. You'll give birth, get into car accidents, pay your bills, or let them pile up. You'll put kids on the school bus, take them out to playdates, wipe their runny noses, take them to the doctor and come home with ten days of gooey pink medicine.

When you're hungry, you'll eat what you choose—even if it's no good for you—or you'll go on a diet. When you're tired, you'll lie down to sleep and dream. You'll wake up in your own bed, in a hotel bed, in your lover's bed, in a stranger's bed. And then you'll go about your day's business; you'll walk out of the bedroom.

You'll go to church. Or you'll avoid it and go somewhere quiet and count your blessings. And one of the blessings you'll count is that you are not in my room.

During the next month or so, I will only leave the isolation room on a stretcher to have total body irradiation, and for no other living reason. The rest of the process of the bone marrow transplant will take place in the room. I will have guests and drugs, constant care and attention. They tell me there will be long stretches with little to do. They tell me I shouldn't expect even to read much. They tell me I'll be lucky to be bored.

Earlier today I had a Hickman catheter surgically inserted into the vena cava, the major vein leading to the heart. Through this port, as they call it, the nurses will give me chemotherapy, and other medicines to alleviate the side effects of chemotherapy, other medicines to fight infections when I have no white count, infusions of red blood and platelets when those counts drop dangerously low, and liter upon liter of salt water to flush down the rest of it. The catheter will let them use my heart as a pump to deliver medicine.

After the catheter was put in, Jane, the intake nurse, told me to go out and have a nice meal, because this will be my last night out for at least two months. Kind of morbid, no? We live in Manhattan, but my wife's father lives in Brookline, five minutes from Dana-Farber. Jean and our two-year-old daughter, Clare, have moved into his apartment for the duration. Our ten-year-old son, Nathan, is here now but will go back to New York and live with our next door neighbors. So this evening we all dutifully went out to my father-in-law's favorite local restaurant. One of Jean's brothers and his girlfriend came too.

Dinner felt like the last meal of a condemned man. Imagine a surprise party where everyone forgets that it is your birthday before you arrive? And they forget the cake. And gifts. Just drinks, and you can't drink tonight.

We sat next to the smokey bar, Clare sound asleep on a pile of coats, Jean and I quiet, the rest talking as cheerily as they could about this and that. Happy banter back and forth, a night on the town, and tomorrow you die. No, tomorrow I go into a room by myself for a month or two, to puke out my guts, to risk death and disability so that for these people I will come out the other end alive and breathing. Better this than cycles of treatments, anxious waiting and watching, and certain recurrence. What did I expect my family to say?

— So long. If we never see you again, it's been grand. Now just in case, we thought tonight we'd help you draft your obit.

But nervous silence would beat nervous chatter. Nathan was happy to joke with his uncle. If I don't make it, he will need his uncle and grandfather all the more. Let them have a laugh. I was speechless. Laughless. I am not a condemned man. I am doing this to live. Celebrate. Tomorrow is the beginning of a life without cancer.

A drink, however much I would have luxuriated in one glass of the finest red on the list, was out of the question. I was told to stop all alcohol a month before I'd be admitted. And the rules for after transplant are more strict. No restaurants, no tap water for a month. No drinks for a year. So Jane told me—Go out tonight and enjoy yourself.

— Enjoy? Really, Jane?

As I was telling myself to stop day dreaming about wine, a cold drip of something fell inside my shirt. What was this? Then another. I looked down inside my shirt. (It was a nice restaurant, not a fancy one.) Couldn't see. I excused myself, and in the not very clean john, stripped to the waist and stared in the mirror at my chest. Blood seeped from under the dressing at the catheter site. I pressed gently on the bandage until the bleeding stopped. Well, dessert was coming. Get me home, and I'll call the hospital.

When we stepped out onto Beacon Street, I breathed very deeply my last draught of fresh cold night air. At least I am going in during the winter. Imagine wasting June in a hospital. What my June will be like is anybody's guess. They tell me most transplant patients wind up back in the hospital sometime or other during the first year out. For the moment I have to worry about January.

Next time you hear from me will be from inside. Now I have to call and find out what the doctor says I should do about my bloody shirt.

DAY MINUS SIX

You can't just walk into your transplant room, dump your bag on the bed and set up shop. You are covered with bugs from home, from the car, from the street. Even, worst of all, bugs from the hospital corridor. These bugs won't normally kill you; they won't even hurt you. They are the regular bugs that everybody breathes, touches, eats everyday. But you are different. Starting tomorrow the staff will begin to wage war on your immune system. In a week, your white blood count will be zilch. Ordinary bugs can be fatal.

So when we arrived on the twelfth floor at Dana-Farber, my nurse, Diana, didn't just open the door and say—In you go, kiddo. First everything we brought for my month's stay had to be rubbed down with a disinfectant and then passed through a double door cubby. All but papers. Reasonably recent books, whatever other evils they may contain, have been found not to carry killer germs. My few clothes we washed the night before, dried on the hottest setting, and stuffed immediately into sealed garbage bags. We didn't have to boil my shirts, just scald them.

Still, Diana wouldn't let me in. This moment I couldn't get in; tomorrow I won't be able to get out. Inside the room, a machine that looked like a large air conditioner on wheels was whirring away, purifying the air. The last occupant in this room was sick. You don't want anything left in the air from her but the crying of her soul's best wishes to survive.

I peered in through the little window. I saw what will become my bed, and thought of the patient who had just gotten out a few days ago, nameless in her suffering. I remembered a day I walked along Eleventh Street in New York by St. Vincent's. The hospital was renovating its insides, and next to the sidewalk stood a dumpster, filled to overflowing with old hospital beds. The load of tangled frames and sagging broken springs screamed. All that suffering and death now gone mute, but for a scraping sound as a frame settled deeper into the dumpster.

"Your room is almost ready. This is what you do next." Diana reminded me I wasn't a visitor; I was expected to do some work here. She talked to me like one of her kids. "You go in. You take off your clothes and put them into one of these garbage bags and take a bath. Howie will get it ready for you." Howie, the nursing assistant, was inside readying the room; he wore the obligatory mask, gloves, and yellow paper gown. He turned off the air machine and wheeled it toward the door. "So you ready?" Diana and Jean had finished wiping down my notebook computer, radio, back roller, and had pushed through the cubby an ambitious pile of books and papers, as if I were coming here because at home I got no peace to work.

"I have to go to the toilet. Should I go before?"

"It's up to you. Doesn't matter."

"In that case, I'll use the toilet on the floor." Here was my condemned man's final wish: pee in a public john.

Relieved, I walked back to my new room, took a deep breath, kissed my wife—"I'm not going anywhere, I'll be in in a minute"—pushed through the door, took off my street clothes, saturated as they were with their street bugs, and plunged into a six inch bath of harsh antibiotic suds.

Jean was waiting for me when I came out of the little bathroom dressed in hospital pj's. Now she wore the mask, gloves, and yellow paper gown. Oy. Kissing is over for this month. Good thing we did it in the corridor. Carpe diem.

Jean went back to her father's after my supper. I'm alone inside the room I won't leave, except to be zapped with radiation, for who knows how long. First off, the place looks like an ordinary hospital private room. A window, a toilet, a bed, curtains, chairs for visitors, a big TV hanging on the wall. Nothing especially high tech, no air lock ante-chamber, no isolation bubble, no air purifier. Just a room, with the door closed. But there are a few other ordinary items you don't expect in a regular private room: a big rack of stainless steal shelving stocked with medical supplies, blood draw supplies, bottles of heparin, saline, and sterile water—all stuff they need to maintain me. A mop and bucket, cleaning rags, my own stethoscope and thermometer so these things won't have to be rubbed clean every time somebody comes to take my temp or mop the floor. There's a balance scale here too. Howie told me that the assistant on night duty has to weigh me first thing in the morning. "They wake me to weigh me?"

"Right, but look, you aren't going to be sleeping more than a few hours at a stretch anyway, so it's no big deal. Pop on the scale, hop back in bed." Hop. Pop. Howie was a small, wiry guy who looked a lot like someone my sister went to high school with. We grew up just outside of Boston, and the nurses and assistants remind me of people I knew in what now seems a previous life.

Diana hitched my Hickman to an IV pump to hydrate me. Tomorrow chemo begins. Tonight is get acquainted time. I wheel my pump to the window.

So this is my view of the world for the next month. I could have had the transplant in New York and looked at the East River, or Seattle and looked at mist, or Houston and looked at a derelict oil well. But here I am in Boston. I haven't lived here in seventeen years, but in view are some very familiar spots: the Beth Israel where my mother was a patient in and out for many years; if I crane my neck, the other way is Mass Mental Health where she worked as a social worker. Boston packs its hospitals in pretty tight. And straight ahead I see a corner of the very hospital I was born in. I'm an elephant come home to die. Well, that is possible, but it's always possible. What do I do with this? Images of coming full circle look an awful lot like standing still, going nowhere, as if life were a giant bungee cord: no matter how far out you stretch it, it will always spring you back where you came from—Don't get uppity sonny, you ain't going nowhere. And kids I went to junior high with are taking care of me. Let me out.

It's not too late, Bob. You haven't taken the treatment yet. You can still pull out. But if you do that, what do you do about the cancer? Talk about coming home to die. You could self-fulfill that one in a hurry. In this room you have a chance. Grab it. Let your mother's haunts be a place of healing. Let the glimpse of where you were born buoy you. Let that baby's mama watch over you. Let me go to sleep already.

DAY MINUS FIVE

Today the bag arrived and treatment started. The bag. Dissolved in saline was an elephantine dose of Cytoxan, a powerful chemotherapy agent. Today is Sunday, and my primary nurse, like most citizens, is off. The substitute nurse is competent but brusk. She has an attitude. She took one look at my vitamin pills and said, "They won't let you take those, I can tell you."

"My transplant doctor said to bring them and see."

"Yeah? Well you can ask the fellow when he comes, but I'd save my breath, if I were you, and chuck them."

She banged around my room, rearranging the furniture and rummaging through the boxes of blood tubes. She gave me a tooth lecture on how I was supposed to clean my teeth with these little sponge-on-the-end-of-a-stick jobs, like flaccid foam tootsie pops. When she said, "I'm not your primary nurse. I'm only here for the day. You probably won't see me again." I heaved a sigh.

First she hooked up an IV bag of mesna, a medicine to protect my bladder from crystals of chemo forming as it left my body later tonight. And another bag of medicine to help reduce nausea. This stuff had worked pretty well when I had outpatient chemotherapy. My smiling nurse told me to forget it. This regime was nothing like anything I had taken on the outside. No way any antiemetic was going to keep me from throwing my guts up into the—"Here, keep this handy"—little blue plastic basin. I asked her if I should eat light this morning, since I'd be seeing my breakfast again later on.

"Oh, you never know," she said. "Might not hit till tonight. Go ahead, eat. For some people it isn't so bad." Talks out of both sides of her mouth, this one does, from years of experience, or is she just a sadist? They all are. Not sadists exactly. The hurt doesn't turn them on so much as the love you show them when they make you feel better. This one can never make me feel better. Not with the shit-eating grin of hers. But never mind her. The bag.

The bag was awful. The bag was filled with poison. The bag—she hung it next to my ear and ran it into the IV machine that had been pumping me full of saline all night—the bag was going to make me sick as hell. I hated that bag. I hated this sour bitch of a nurse for connecting my catheter to pure evil and letting this clear innocuous-looking filth drip slowly into my vena cava. I squirmed in my chair. The fellow, the nurse, Jean, all stood dumb watching the dripping, and I, like a child, looked up in faint hope, turning from one face to another and then back to the dripping fluid. Poison, straight up, no chaser.

This bag of piss, this condensed, dissolved horror, was the very best chance—my Sloan-Kettering oncologist, Ken Offit, claimed the only chance—to save my life. And I loved it. Forget that each drop I would pay for; every drop that went into me was another moment, another chance, another beat for life. And I sat up straight and took a deep breath and welcomed it into my body. I'm not a praying man, but I blessed the Cytoxan as it dripped into me. "Do your thing," was all I could lamely articulate through tears. I imagined that the chemo went in and right through me, dragging, pulling, pushing the lymphoma out with it.

And believe me, tonight something has started coming out. Keep that basin handy, here we go. What an awful mess this is. The surface of the hospital is scrubbed clean. But on any other level—the microbial, the emotional, the intestinal—it is one god-awful churning mess. Think of the plumbing. I do what I do, the nursing assistant measures and flushes it. We think it's gone. But it lingers in the pipes, in the twists and turns of the traps. The red sharps bucket, with its biohazard symbol, looks neat and crisp; inside is a bloody mess of needles, tubing, and wipes.

Behind my visitors masks, gloves, and robes, behind their kind and encouraging words, lurks all measure of fear, horror, pity, and deep thanks that it's me in the bed, not them, and the guilt that goes with the thanks. And beneath my one-step-at-a-time coping, lurks anger and profound loathing. Why else do I accuse a perfectly well-intentioned nurse of being a sadist? And something else I can't name that comes from growing up with my mother's cancer and turning around and living it out, this time in my own body. More, if I can, on that one later. Now excuse me. I have to throw up.

DAY MINUS FOUR

The night is long but not a horror. The night nurse gave me Ativan, a sedative, which knocked me out, but now I'm awake and can't get back to sleep. The nausea they pretty well have under control. The vomiting goes on. It comes on suddenly. A bell rings somewhere in my nervous nervous system and up I chuck. Keep that basin handy. Like any teenager, when I learned to drink, I threw up a lot. A few beers would make me sick, and bingo. Like this, only by the end of the next day I was sober. The chemo and the antiemetics make me woozy. The nurse told me it will get worse. How much worse we'll see. But this I can take, if this is it, which I doubt. You can take just about anything for a couple of days. We have barely started here. I get another bag of the Cytoxan later this morning and then three days of total body irradiation. They say the radiation will destroy anything left of my digestive track. They tell me to be prepared to sit on the toilet with my intestines pouring out one end while I puke into the basin whatever hasn't reached the intestines from the other end.

Chemo attacks rapidly dividing cells wherever they are: mouth, guts, hair, or cancer. The most noticeable side effects last a couple of weeks. The worst is not the puking and shitting, it's the fatigue, which can last months. And worse than that, they tell me—the real danger starting when all my white blood cells are gone—is infection. This whole business is barbaric. When they find out how to re-order genes and really rid people of their cancers, we will look back—those of us left standing—on bone marrow transplants as the dark ages. But I could die waiting for the cure. My mother did, though she stuck it out for twenty-two years of breast cancer treatment, remission, relapse, and metastasis. Wait, here comes my new nurse. I'll be back.

She's lovely. I asked her if she would be my primary nurse, meaning: Are you assigned to be my nurse? But she thought I meant: Will you please be my nurse? Someone forgot to tell me I have a voice in this decision. Never mind, Sandy is wonderful, a large woman with a twinkle in her eye and what seems today to be constant good humor. And she is pregnant. She's bringing two of us into a new world, and those hormones are keeping her buoyant. She is lovely, lovely and spirited. Working with transplant patients she must long ago have learned to take a deep breath in the corridor and put on the smile. Of course I can't see her smile under the mask, but it's there. I see it in her eyes, and as her mask inches up her nose when I manage to say something funny. Maybe hers isn't such a bad job after all. Transplant patients, as sick as we get, have not come here to die. Sandy is not maintaining us in our last days. We are going through all this in hope of beating the cancer. This has to make an enormous difference to a nurse.

When I was taking outpatient chemotherapy at Sloan-Kettering, I got to know my chemo nurse pretty well. She always asked me for the latest test results and what the doctors were telling me. We talked about our families, bike riding, her employer, my doctor. One day, after I said something like—Who knows if all this is doing any good—she leaned over very close (three other patients were in the room) and whispered, "You're beating this sucker." Into the ground, Elizabeth. Deep into the ground. The doctors here probably won't let people into their study—even people with a good chance of benefiting—if we don't believe in our own chances.

They let me in because I had a lot of disease, but localized in the lungs; because they thought they had a chance of doing me some good; because I was otherwise healthy; because I had family support; because I was referred by a doctor they knew; because I'm relatively young at forty-four. And, though no one dares say this, maybe because I'm insured; because I'm an educated, smarter than average white guy whom they can talk to; because I appeared to listen carefully and ask questions; because I've been working my tail off to get good care.

But about a month ago, as we waited for me to recover from the last outpatient chemo cycle, they suddenly got me scared that they wouldn't take me. I thought the choice was mine if I wanted to go through with it. Transplant is an enormous undertaking. They've told me I'll be a year recovering with only a fifty-fifty chance of getting rid of the disease. Not everyone survives transplant or the period of recovery. I'm taking a big risk here. I was frightened and angry that I would have to give it so much time. I had my doubts. What if the thing does me no good? I'll spend my little time puking in the hospital instead of . . . instead of what? I was going to be happy on the beach knowing a stone was left unturned?

One evening, Lini Pandite, my transplant doctor here, called to say she wanted me to fax her some recent test results from Sloan-Kettering. She had to present my case to a committee before we could go ahead. Wasn't the choice mine? Now there was a committee. What committee? Who were they to make this choice for me?

We don't have a fax machine in our three room West Side apartment—we really don't have space for ourselves—so I walked to a copy store that drizzly December night. When I got halfway across Broadway, I stopped on the traffic island waiting for the light to change and started to cry. I want this transplant. In the moment I was more frightened of losing the chance than I was of the procedure. How dare some committee take this away from me? If they rejected me, I'd have to start looking for another hospital. I already had a doctor at Farber I liked. I put a lot of effort into getting ready for Farber. I was horrified by the prospect of starting all over somewhere else.

I waited a few tense days until I heard again from Dr. Pandite. Everything was in order to go ahead. She didn't bring up the committee business, except to report that the chief of the service asked what she was waiting for.

I took the first bag of chemo yesterday. There is no turning back. I made my choice, and my choice will make me.

Sandy has hung bag two. I am woozy from the meds and my eyes don't focus well. No doctor is in the room this time; now the deal is routine. I watch the poison drip. I remember yesterday, mumble the little blessing again just in case, and close my eyes. Bag two is also bag last. No more chemotherapy. Tomorrow begins three days of radiation. The next bag of stuff they drip into me will be my bone marrow, the beginning of my rescue. But no jumping ahead. No step left out. Every moment suffered, endured, overcome. OK, not every moment. Pass the Ativan please.

DAY MINUS THREE

They're coming to take me for the first of six radiation treatments. Farber doesn't have the machine to give total body irradiation, so they have to truck me to Brigham and Women's Hospital. OK with me. But they won't let me just walk across the street; that might be easy and even pleasant, but dangerous. They take me by ambulance. Now I'm dressed in a clean johnny, robe, paper gown, gloves, and mask—like my visitors—and pacing while I wait for the crew to show up. I've seen where they are taking me; a month ago when I met the radiation oncologist, I was shown the radiation room. A kind of de-mystery tour.

Later: I'm back from the first TBI treatment. The route there is almost comical. After I'm all dressed—there are throwaway slippers too—Sandy opens the door and I sit on a gurney. She and Kathy wrap me head to foot in blankets. Only my eyes are uncovered. Then our entourage heads for the back elevator—five of us: Sandy, a nursing assistant, one of the ambulance paramedics, a security guard, and me, the patient patient. The guard's job is to clear the hallway between my room and the elevator, lock the elevator so that it won't stop on any intermediate floor, and then keep the way clear until I'm loaded into the back of the ambulance. Everybody wears masks, gloves, and gowns. Jean can't come with this time because there isn't room in the ambulance. For the next five trips, Sandy will be out, and Jean can take her place.

The whole thing smacks of high security, as if I'm a political candidate or some pasha. But I'm just me, a forty-four-year-old father of two from New York, a freelance theatrical lighting designer and sometime writer come back to my birthplace to try to live a little longer, and not die from cancer or from the treatment of cancer. I accept that I have to be wrapped like a mummy and carried to and from the X-ray machine and that the radiation will make me very sick, that I will be miserable before I'm better because nothing comes cheap and easy. I'm going under before passing over to the side of health and life. I didn't choose cancer, but I choose the heart with which to fight cancer. It may be that I carry cancer genes. It may be that my mother's history, getting breast cancer when I was six and our living with it for twenty-two years, proved that cancer is something you live with, that it was, in this child's eyes, normal. But how I deal with it now is a new, not-normal business. Whether the doctors will save me or not, I am here facing what has to be faced with my nearsighted, now drugged eyes as open as I can get them. Or so I wish to think.

After they put me into the ambulance, where do we go? Across the street, literally from one driveway to another. I can see the Brigham from my room. Not just see the building, I can look into rooms across the way and see people moving around. When we arrive, bells go off, their security guard clears the corridor, and I'm pushed down the hall and delivered to the radiation chamber.

The room is ordinary. The machine is not threatening looking or dangerous or hateful. It's a table. A kind of mesh trampoline surface that the technician has me lie on facing the contraption overhead. Last month when I visited, she explained that the thing zaps the patient all over from both sides at once, which is why the table isn't solid under me; there's another radiator under there. This is supposed to make the zapping easier for the patient because you don't have to flip over to be charred on the other side. Cooks in half the time, like having the oven and broiler on at the same time and really roasting your steak. For some people lying still is a problem. Lie still I can do. I can dream and drift and meditate. The recipe calls for twenty minutes per side, but only a total of twenty on Brigham's special rotisserie. To be out of the isolation room an extra twenty minutes wouldn't have been a bad thing at all. No choice. Take the faster machine and love it. Love it to bits.

The tech carefully positions me under the monster and, over and under my chest, places lead shields that had been specially cast for me a month ago. The lungs are sensitive and need to be protected from radiation. Odd in my case since the disease was seen only in the lungs. They said I needed the shields anyway, and they couldn't vary the protocol or the study results would be worthless. And wherever the disease is, if the radiation could damage the lungs even more than they already are, there is no point in exposing them.

I have to trust that I put myself in good hands. Everyone has told me they don't know exactly what will happen after they treat me. They aren't sure because they never are and because this particular presentation of this disease is rare. Every step of the way coming into transplant a doctor has said—We do this and we see what happens, and if X happens we do Y, but if X doesn't happen we do Z. And so on. When, last month, I talked to the radiation oncologist, this nice, unassuming, even bashful guy whom I never met before and haven't seen since, said quietly, "Look, we know if you don't have the transplant, the disease will come back, no matter what we treat you with." He sounded pretty convincing to me.

Once she had me properly positioned on the trampoline, the tech asked for my tape. I was told to bring music, so I did what I was told. I brought Bach, the English Suite that I heard late at night in the hospital a year and a half ago. The tech told me to lie still, and just as she left the room she popped the tape in. I didn't need it. The boom box makes terrible sound, and I would prefer the machine noise, my breathing, and my thoughts. Never mind. Do what I'm told. They'll worry about me without the music, even if my taste is a little precious. Let the bad sound go. Too late to get up and change it now. Get zapped.

There is no pain with the radiation, no sensation at all. And that, when you think about it, is scary. The radiation oncologist told me that TBI will almost certainly leave me sterile. But in the chamber, I try not to scare myself with these thoughts. I close my eyes and listen to Bach. Tomorrow, Charlie Parker, then maybe some Mozart. Until then . . .

DAY MINUS TWO

After TBI treatment we do the whole rigmarole in reverse to get me back into the room. Sandy reminds me to strip off the hospital pj's and bathe because we don't know what kind of bugs I might have picked up on my outing.

While bathing I have to be careful of the lumens on the Hickman line. I'm not supposed to let the tubes, set deep into the vena cava under my collarbone, get wet, so I tape them high on the shoulder. The tubes are called ports, as if I'm a boat or a computer. An in/out port. Medicine and saline go in, and blood comes out for testing. Later I will have to be transfused through these ports. I may have to be fed through them if I can't keep anything down or develop terribly painful mouth sores. The bandage that covers the entry site has to be changed every third day. Sandy does it now, but she is going to teach me how, and then I'm responsible. Like my teeth. Everybody has a job to do here. No shirking. No malingering.

I'm still getting used to this place. This is my home. I can't tell you I'm claustrophobic or that I hate the place or this is even the last place in the world you'd want to be. There are worse places. You don't want to be in Bosnia, although you could survive that war and have no cancer. You don't want to be on death row. You don't want to be living on the street, not in January in Boston. But you don't want to be here. We put up photos of the kids. And some of Clare's drawings. I brought a few books, but have barely looked at them. I brought paper and pencils, but the tape recorder is all I can manage right now. I've asked friends to send snapshots of themselves instead of cards. They think I'm strange—But hey, whatever you want; better you than me. You don't want to be here. The photos and drawings don't make me cry anymore. They've become wall paper. All these people on the outside going about their business. Me in here. Pisses me off. Jean's been the only visitor so far. They call. They complain about the weather. It snows. It's cold. They tell me I picked a good time to be indoors for a month. They tell me I'm better off inside. Bull. I am not well off. Or am I? In a good hospital with people who know what they are doing and care. I couldn't be better. I have something my callers don't. I have a chance today and tomorrow and for the next however long it takes to fight the thing that could kill me.

When I talked about death, people would respond with some version of—Any of us crossing the street could be hit by a bus. I'd respond—Yeah, but when I get to the other side of the street I will still have cancer. What I'm doing here is trying to let the bus hit the cancer, but to jump my self out of the way at the last second. Jump too soon and the cancer jumps with me. Jump too late . . .

Later they will come and take me back to the radiation chamber for my second dose and do the whole thing over again. They have to split up my dosage into six sessions over three days. One humongous dose would be too much for me all at once. Jump.

DAY MINUS ONE

Six a.m. Last TBI today. Routine. Throwing up is routine. I keep the basin always at hand. I feel queazy all the time, but the violent nausea comes on quickly and then it's gone. Up I chuck and I'm done. The nurse gives me a push of trilathon, an antiemetic and sedative. I'm getting spacey. I'm uncomfortable but not horribly so. I brought a mat into the room, and I try to get down on it in the morning and stretch for forty-five minutes. I'm not going anywhere, so I can take leisurely time with yoga. At home I'm always rushed, here—No problem mon, you got all day, relax, be easy. Be happy—Except that these three days of TBI I have to finish the yoga by ten so they can ship me back to the radiation box. What a schedule.

The night nursing assistant wakes me at six to weigh me. They need to know how much weight I'm puking and shitting off. But why six? It must be one of the last tasks for the night shift. Take temperature, blood pressure, pulse, weigh 'em, and go home. Mildred, one of the regular night nurses, always looks very tired. For some family reason, Mildred has to work nights, but it isn't good for her. She never seems to be able to open her eyes all the way, and her eyes are all I see of her face. Mildred may be suffering from sleep deprivation, but I think she is depressed. And she's the nurse. So what? Mildred, if she has to be, can be depressed. She does her work well enough. I don't talk to her much after she gives me the Ativan, which lets me get some sleep without puking. And Mildred is an angel in the night when I need anything. I love her even for being depressed. People can get too cheery around here. I love Sandy too, but she's decided the way to go is cheery. Up. An upper this place isn't.

People will say Mildred is entitled to be depressed because she works with very sick cancer patients, who themselves must be depressed. This place may not be bubbly, but really it is not depressing. Giving up is depressing. Here we are fighting for our lives. Mildred helps. What could be depressing about that? So I think her glum effect has its source elsewhere. Mildred should find a baby sitter and work days.

The other regular night nurse is Larry. If Larry is depressed he does a much better job hiding it. Larry is a hoot. He brightens my otherwise dark night, even when he sneaks into my room trying not to wake me.

"When do you want your Ativan?" he asked last night.

"Well I don't know, maybe tonight I don't need it."

"You want my opinion? OK, I know you didn't ask for it. Take the drugs. If you don't need them, who the hell does?"

Suppertime. Another day of snow. The last trip to Brigham's was a joke. They got me down as far as the loading ramp but couldn't back the ambulance into the door because of all the snow. Cars, ambulances, and delivery trucks were sliding all over the place. Another ambulance was stuck in the loading zone. First they wheeled me back inside while the drivers tried to get the crippled ambulance jimmied out of the way. They must have moved it some, because the paramedics wheeled me back out into the slush. Then everything ground to a halt. Some other vehicle was stuck. Drivers, security guys, paramedics slid back and forth hollering and waving their arms.

But I was in heaven. To be wrapped tight and warm and to be left alone in the cold air, so fresh compared with the hot hospital air of the last week, was glorious. I gulped down as much as I could of this free outside, the normal air you and everybody else breathes. This was cheating. I wasn't supposed to be here. Really, the whole deal with switching hospitals for forty minutes was already questionable. And then to be left alone while they tried to figure out how to get the ambulance twenty feet closer was a riot. I didn't even mind the smell of ambulance exhaust. To play hookey, to be out in the fresh of it—Ahhhh.

Finally they gave up on backing the ambulance into the door, and wheeled me out across the slushy driveway and into the waiting wagon. Even in the snow, an ambulance ride across the street took almost no time.

My last TBI ended to Exultate Jubilate on the boom box, not exactly the sound quality of the angels, but, hallelujah, the end has come. No more treatments. I have received a nearly lifetime sterilizing dose of radiation. They can't do this to me again.

As the paramedic wheeled me out, the radiation technician handed me my Mozart tape, and, wrapped in a rubber glove, the four lead shields she had put over my lungs to protect them during TBI.

"Here, these belong to you," she said. "They won't fit anybody else."

"Melt them down. Start over," I said. But I took them.

"Good luck," she said, and patted my blankets. The shields were small and heavy and each one had my name written on tape stuck to the back. What am I going to do with these? A souvenir. Don't let me say Brigham never gave me anything.

One other gift they gave me. The day I went in for the bone marrow harvest, they gave me a canvas Brigham and Women's tote bag to put my street clothes into overnight. I am having an autologous bone marrow transplant. This means that the doctors are using my own bone marrow, which they extracted—they use the faintly barbarous word "harvest"—then treated, and froze. They can do this because I have never shown disease in the bone marrow. People whose disease shows up extensively in the marrow must have an allogeneic transplant, bone marrow from a donor. Allogeneic transplants, even with matching marrow from a family member, are more dangerous. With donor marrow there is the risk that the patient's immune system will reject the marrow as a foreign invader.

My oncologist at Memorial Sloan-Kettering wanted Farber to harvest my marrow months ago, even before we decided definitely to go for the transplant.

"The worst thing that can happen is your marrow rots in Boston," he said.

But Farber will not store the marrow, especially without the certainty that the patient will transplant. They want fresh marrow. The harvest was done three weeks ago. I went in early in the morning; they put me under general anesthesia, and, through twelve punctures in my pelvis, sucked about a liter of bloody marrow. The procedure took about an hour and a half they tell me. I wasn't there. My tush was, but I have no memory. I do have twelve scars. I stayed overnight in the hospital while they transfused me with the blood separated from the marrow.

The next morning on the breakfast tray, with the OJ and the oatmeal, was a cheeky note thanking me for what I had done. I was very generous and I should go out and treat myself. I deserved it. Did I say cheeky note? I stared at the paper for a long time. Maybe I was still anesthetized, but what could this mean? Why this moment to give myself a treat? What was generous about having my bone marrow removed so I could have it transplanted back to me? Then I saw. The note was for donors, not patients having autologous transplants. They got me mixed up with someone else. Or maybe they only had one note for everybody, and if autologous patients didn't already know what they were here for, then a confusing note at breakfast wouldn't hurt them. Once I got back into my street clothes, the nurse, with offhanded grace, told me I could keep the tote bag. Hooray. This will come in handy, especially if they have to transplant me again.

For a cancer patient, a bone marrow transplant isn't done so much because you have lousy marrow and need new, like a kidney transplant. In order to destroy your disease, the doctors give you such massive doses of chemotherapy and radiation that, in the meantime, they destroy your bone marrow. Transplant really means rescue. Without it you die. The lengthy consent form I signed allowed me to pull out at any time before the first dose of chemo. After that, anything but following the strict protocol would likely mean death.

When the marrow left Brigham's, it was hand carried to Dana-Farber's lab. Everybody asks, "What happens if it gets mixed up with somebody else's?" To guard against that possibility, they do only one harvest a day. Everything is triple checked. Still—What if? They say there is no if. After the harvest, the marrow is treated. Farber uses a special monoclonal antibody to seek out cancer cells. Even though none of my bone marrow biopsies showed lymphoma, the disease is considered systemic, and if the doctors reinfused untreated marrow, they would likely give me back my disease. And even with the treatment, everything by the book, the chances of my being disease free in five years are only fifty-fifty. Better than nothing. But still a long shot.

When I got back to the room from the last radiation, I bathed and threw up. Now there is no telling when next I'll pass through that door.

But I do know the next step in the process. Treatment is over; nothing more to hurt my marrow, so tomorrow I get it back. Why wait? Shit, I hope they give me the right bag. Don't worry about it now. I've stepped so deeply into it, there's nothing left to do but keep my head up and not wiggle further into doubt and muck.

DAY ZERO

All morning I waited anxiously for my marrow. I did the yoga, bathed, Sandy changed the dressing on my Hickman site. Jean took Clare to day care and came straight to the hospital to be here when the marrow arrived. When it did, the attending physician, the fellow, the intern, and Sandy came with it. The intern tacked a plastic bag with a syringe in it onto the bulletin board at the foot of my bed, and in the pass-through appeared a breathing bag.

Everybody was quiet and seemed pretty relaxed as Sandy hung the bag of marrow and attached it to the IV pump. Such a big deal, months spent trying to decide the best treatment and choose the hospital, but here this morning, it all came to a head in about forty uneventful minutes. The reinfusion of the marrow is just like a blood transfusion.

Myth has it that the marrow circulates through the blood stream and finds its way back inside the bones where it belongs. I was Hansel and Gretel looking for a way out of the forest, and the 500cc of yellow pudding-looking stuff in the IV bag was my bread crumbs. I took a deep breath. Find your way home. Come back to me. I am home.

I sat in the only comfortable chair. Everybody else stood and watched, nonchalantly chatting but all the while watching me. A patient can have a sudden and violent reaction, though for most the process is as benign as it was for me. Just one more bag of fluid—this one the most expensive bag you can imagine. I tasted something funny and that was it. They say that you can tell a patient who has just gotten his bone marrow because the room smells of garlic from something in the preservative used in storing the marrow. I couldn't smell it. They could.

I tried to muster some appropriate enthusiasm for the fact of the event—this is the end of cancer treatment, the beginning of a life without cancer—but the reality of the moment, a simple infusion, lacked drama. Until the bag was running down to empty. Then I felt a lightness, a tingling in the chest. And the assembled company felt something too because their chatter turned genuinely lighthearted. I sat up straighter. I felt in my chest the lightness of laughter. If I were going to stop breathing, I would have done that by now. Tick off another step to health. I joined in their lightness as best I could. Yes, oh yes.

More difficulty is to come. The most dangerous period, when my blood counts will drop to nothing, is still ahead. There is a lag between the treatment and when the circulating blood cells all die. By early next week I should have no counts left. There's another lag between the infusion of the marrow and when it begins to produce blood cells. We were by no means out of the woods, perhaps even deeper into it. But I could smell the bread crumbs, and right this moment I had my marrow back, and right this moment I faced no more treatment, and right this moment I felt light enough to float to the ceiling. Not giddy or high, but light. Well, I'd been puking my guts out, shitting buckets, losing weight, losing every hair, no wonder I felt light.

When the last of my marrow was on its way back to where it belonged, and I was still breathing and my heart was still pumping, they left Jean and me to ourselves.

Surely they had warned her in graphic and specific terms what might have happened. The syringe on the bulletin board was filled with epinephrine. They probably told her that if I stopped breathing they'd have to shove her out of the room and that she should go fast when told. But none of that happened.

We smiled, hugged, and sighed a long well-at-least-that's-over-and-done-with sigh. Then I threw up.

DAY ONE

Mildred smelled the garlic. She passed in and out of my room many times last night to check my toilet and my temp, pulse, and blood pressure. I don't sleep very soundly here, and we talked now and then.

"How you doing tonight, Mildred?" The sad-eyed lady looked less depressed in the dark.

"You got your marrow back today," she said.

"I don't get to have a secret, huh?"

"Here? A medical secret? Smelling like that? Unlikely. Try to get some sleep. You have a long haul yet."

The lymphoma that landed me here had been a secret for no one knows how long. I was diagnosed a year ago—and a long year it's been—with a low-grade non-Hodgkin's lymphoma presenting only in the lungs. But the lungs were one-third full of the stuff. The disease was not caught early, which was as much of a blow as the diagnosis. I thought I was a healthy, aware guy who would at least be careful and find out early. But no. I had the lymphoma for a long time, years; maybe five, maybe more. Low grade means slow growing, which is good in that it doesn't kill you right away, and not good because it is incurable by conventional treatments. Even this bone marrow transplant gives me only half a chance of being disease free in five years. Fifty-fifty is better than no chance. I said that before? You'll hear it again.

A year and a half ago I came down with mycoplasma pneumonia. At least that's what the chest X-ray, CT, and blood tests showed. I was treated with high-dose antibiotics in the hospital for a week and outpatient for three weeks. But when the X-ray didn't clear, my doctors began other tests. The internist, Richard Collens, and the pulmonary specialist he sent me to, Mary O'Sullivan, were wonderful. They wouldn't leave me alone when I kept asking what would be the harm in giving it another couple of weeks because I was sure I'd get better. The doctors had a piece of hard evidence in the X-ray, and felt obliged to press forward. I had pulmonary function tests that showed I had lost about a third of my lung capacity. They say you have more capacity than you use, but looking back I knew that I had had a few experiences of shortness of breath on exertion, bicycling and backpacking uphill. I chalked it up to age. I'm forty-four. But Richard, bless his heart, looked at me as if I were joking. Something was the matter here.

A year ago December, Mary O'Sullivan did a bronchoscopy, which involves putting a tube into the windpipe and looking around inside the lungs. The thing has a little camera on the end, and I looked up from the table and saw my insides on TV. It looked like a pink subway tunnel in there. The bronchoscope also allows her to take small biopsies of the lung.

The first biopsy result told her that I had something called lymphocytic interstitial pneumonitis, LIP, a kind of autoimmune disease. That news was a shock. She had thought I had BOOP, bronchiolitis obliterans organizing pneumonia, something that can happen after a bout of pneumonia. Both are treated with corticosteroids, but LIP does not have a good prognosis. She said young people—for this purpose I was considered young—do better with the treatment. OK, when do we start.

Mary said she couldn't start until they ruled out lymphoma, which absolutely had to be done before this diagnosis was accepted. "Yeah, but in the meantime, why not treat as if it's LIP?" I asked. "If I respond, then it's LIP."

"No, no. That would be a terrible mistake because the lymphoma would appear to respond to the treatment but would not be dealt with in a meaningful way. You have to have an open lung biopsy."

She sent me to a surgeon who explained that he would perform a thoracotomy and all that that entailed. He would cut my chest wide open and take out some really juicy samples of tissue called wedges. He would also go after some lymph nodes hiding behind my breast bone. Recovery time—six weeks. And he said he wouldn't fix anything for me. Just answer some questions for my doctors. Scared the living shit out of me.

In the meantime I was sent to a hematologist. He looked at the tests so far and said, "I will be surprised and educated, if it turns out you have lymphoma." So, OK, maybe the surgery will be good news. But before the surgery, he recommended that the biopsy slides from the bronchoscopy be taken up to a lab at Columbia for more careful study by a world renowned pathologist. Imagine me clutching my precious little slides on the uptown subway. Later I learned that this hemato-pathologist was the kind of world famous that no one at Dana-Farber was likely to contradict.

I didn't know what to wish for. As Jean pointed out, he couldn't prove a negative. If the pathologist didn't see lymphoma in the tiny scrap of flesh Mary O'Sullivan snipped out of my lung, that would only have meant he didn't see it, not that it wasn't there. Then the big surgery would be a must. The only way to avoid surgery was for him to come up with a diagnosis of lymphoma. I knew if I had to have lymphoma, I didn't want both it and the thoracotomy. What to wish for?

Word came in phone call. Not from the pathologist or Mary O'Sullivan, but from Richard Collens. He was pretty shaken up actually and very sad. He gave me all the time I needed on the phone. Why wasn't I floored by the news, devastated, burned up?

I do not know. You aren't going to believe it, but I was somewhat relieved. The question of what was the matter with my lungs had been dragging on for five months. Finally we had a diagnosis. "At least the mystery is over," I said, almost to comfort Richard. Pretty weird.

And what I now have isn't some obscure lung ailment, LIP. I had called the big expert "who wrote the chapter" on LIP, a doctor in Colorado. He told me he was following twenty-five patients. Cancer is an enormous medical establishment. And ordinary people know about it. My family wouldn't say—Huh, what's LIP? They would know immediately this was serious business.

"So we meet again," said the hematologist, "and I am indeed educated. I've searched the literature and the NCI database and have not come up with one case similar to yours." Was I supposed to be proud of my unique status, or scared shitless that no one would know what to do with me?

He took a bone marrow biopsy: done under a local anesthetic, he shoved a big needle into the back of my pelvic bone. "You have very hard bones," he said as he rocked back and forth to get the needle in. Should I be proud or annoyed? After the procedure, he said, "You have a high tolerance for pain. That's good." I got this cue; now I am supposed to feel proud. But he was looking much farther down the cancer treatment road than I was at the moment.

He proposed to treat me with nine cycles of CHOP chemotherapy. Who knew, without another such case on record, maybe this plan would cure me. Hmmm.

And here I am in the ultimate big deal of medicine. After I had a second opinion from Sloan-Kettering, I called the hematologist back and told him they had recommended a bone marrow transplant. He said he would have gotten around to it if the CHOP didn't work. "I think it's premature. But consider transplant if you want the best 1993 has to offer."

"Oh, I see," I said. Seeing nothing. Why the hell wouldn't I want the best 1993 had to offer. Why on earth would I want less? Why was he prepared to offer less? But I see it now that I am here finding out first hand what he was saving to talk about later. Mary O'Sullivan was shocked that Memorial had suggested right off the bat to go for the transplant. "Bone marrow transplantation is an enormous undertaking." You can say that again, Mary. And at first I was not sold on it by any means.

Liza, a nursing assistant, comes to check my temp and output. At other hospitals the nursing assistants fill your pitcher of ice water in the night. Here I can only drink bottled sterile water. If I want it cold, I have to keep it in the fridge and get it myself. I miss the comforting sound of the ice tinkling in the pitcher when they wake me. In order for the assistant to see what I did in the toilet, she has to turn on the light in the john. She never turns it off. As long as I can walk and pee standing up, I refuse to keep the urinal hanging on the bed rail. I know the room well enough to walk to the john in the semi-darkness, and holding the jug with one hand and lifting my johnny with the other, pee like an almost normal man. I can do the whole thing without touching myself, so I don't have to wash my hands, which along with turning on the light will wake me up. I have asked that the assistants turn off the light when they are finished measuring my turd, but they never remember. So I have to switch the light off before I open the bathroom door or risk lying awake for an hour. Why is this my job? Why can't they remember? I'll put up a sign, which they'll have to turn on the light to read, smarty.

My mind is racing and I won't get back to sleep. Sleep is so important here, but I'm too tired right now to talk about it.

I'll tell you later. Good night. Well 'night anyway.

DAY TWO

Sleep is crucial. Yes, I am sick to my stomach and sick in the basin and in the "hat" resting in the toilet mouth. But the fatigue is like nothing else I have ever experienced. All the time. I wake up tired. Used to be I'd put in a tough week of long hours in the theater and on tour, and one good night's sleep would get me going again. But now nothing relieves the fatigue. The yoga I do every morning is very gentle but leaves me bushed. Jello lunch makes me tired. Going to and from the bathroom wears me out.

When I first wake up, I'm not sure if I'm asleep or awake. I'm a lump filling the bed. The body sends no signals of alertness; my skin doesn't tingle or itch; my muscles don't ache to stretch. I lie perfectly still for a long time until I know that what I'm seeing is not dreaming.

I know because I do not dream about the hospital. Victor Frankel reported that concentration camp inmates did not dream about the camp until after they were liberated. In the camp they dreamed of food. Their dreams fed them. If I see the bed, the pictures my daughter drew, photos of family, the one-date-per-page calendar—each morning I rip off another day survived—the chart telling how low my blood counts are falling, the balance scale on which each morning we measure how much weight I'm dropping, the little fridge we keep the jello I try bravely not to throw up, the mercifully blank TV—this stuff tells me my eyes must be open. It takes twenty minutes to raise enough energy to crawl out of bed.

But I can't tell you what a savior sleep is. Sleep is travel. I get out of this room. I roam. I am away from cancer, from bone marrow transplant, from hospital. Where do I go? Places. Without remembering a dream, I wake with the sense that I've been somewhere. I'd love to tell you that in my dream I cruised the Alaska coast and saw icebergs calve from glaciers. Or that I returned to the wild Maine island that was the base camp for the canoe trips I took as a kid. But I have nothing so neat to report. All I know is that I was away from my desk, out to lunch, absent.

But one dream repeats. In it I am in bed in a second story alcove, a kind of large bay window. Outside it is a sunny May morning, the trees are in leaf and whispering in the breeze, new leaves not tough enough yet to rustle. The windows are open and the morning air cools the sheets. That's it. I like to guess somebody is in bed with me and that soon we will get up and go outside together. We'll swim or run and suck in great lungs-full of fresh morning. But so far all that I know is that the room is cool, the windows are open, and the leaves are moving in the sunlight. Stay tuned.

DAY THREE

Today my counts dropped to nothing. No cells being made. I will have transfusions of red cells and platelets and they have already started giving me G-mcsf to stimulate the white cells as soon as the marrow engrafts. When I have no platelets, Sandy won't let me do my yoga even. Some vessel breaks inside and I more or less bleed to death. At least that's what she implied.

I should call Dr. Offit. But what will I say. Hello from the hell you put me in? Even the bad news phone call with Richard Collens was not as anxiety producing as my first afternoon at Sloan-Kettering when I went for a second opinion.

Dr. Offit is distantly related. Through a series of phone calls to relatives, my father was led to him. I had just been diagnosed. It was good for him to help in a concrete way. Offit talked to me from his home at night. I told him what I knew from the path report and from what Mary and the hematologist had said and how I was feeling. He told me to get all the films, slides, and reports, and submit them before our appointment in a week. "You'll see," he said, "getting all this stuff together will be a job. Do it. Tomorrow call my secretary, tell her I told you to make an appointment for the 23rd. She won't want to do it because I'm teaching then and not seeing patients. But push and tell her I said so. When was your last chest X-ray?"

"After the bronchoscopy."

"No, I mean before all this."

"I don't know. College. Twenty years ago."

"See if you can get it. It would be interesting to compare.

Good luck. You'll need it."

He was right. It was a major job getting all the films and slides and the paraffin block and all the reports. Most of the stuff came from Mary O'Sullivan, but she was overworked with no assistant in sight.

I dug deep into my files and came up with my old student ID number and called University Hospital in Madison. The number was magic. Within a minute, the woman on the other end had the date and time of the X-ray, January, 1970, more than twenty years ago. In Wisconsin I still existed. That was a relief. To get the report I would have to write a letter, but she was sure the film itself was long since destroyed. I'd take what I could get. Report came back: chest normal. Marginally useless information. Also in the medical record was treatment for a bat bite. Now this truly is another story, but the experience of waking up in the middle of the night with a bat crawling in the bed came crashing back through an intern's scratchy handwriting. I can only hope to be around to look at Sandy's notes in twenty years.

Of course I arrived early for the appointment at Memorial and of course I had to wait. Memorial waiting areas are modern snazzy compared to the nineteenth-century gentility of St. Luke's. The place is like a nice hotel, not too too expensive, but real plants, incandescent lighting, framed art prints, fresh paint.

I waited.

A young woman in a long blue coat told me Dr. Offit would be delayed. I could go to the cafeteria if I wanted. No, I'd wait here and pretend to read. Dark blue coats are session assistants, young hospital administrators in grad-school training. Light blue jackets are volunteers. Brownish green is for maintenance. Doctors, nurses, technicians wear white coats, like they are supposed to. Hospital policy. At Farber some of the doctors don't bother with coats of any color. And when they come to see me, they look like everybody else in yellow paper gowns and masks.

Finally she came back and took me to an exam room. And I waited. The room was spare but efficient: desk, two chairs and a sort of bench, an exam table, a supply cabinet. Nathan was at home now by himself. Jean was upstate teaching. I had been waiting an hour. There was a phone on the desk. I called him. He was worried. I had told him the appointment would run long, but he had to go to a choral recital and was worried I wouldn't make it in time to take him. "How can it take much longer? He'll come soon, and we'll talk, and I'll come home."

"Just come as soon as you can, Dad."

I waited.

Offit's fellow, Dr. Rubin, came to take a history. As part of the mound of papers and films I had submitted, I wrote a chronology of the illness so far. Rubin had read it and said, "You've done a pretty good job here, but I'll just go through it with you, see if you left anything out." Then he proceeded to read back to me what I had written, underlining as he went. I elaborated here and there, and got confused once or twice about whose role was whose. When he finished my dissertation, he stood up and said he would come back later when Dr. Offit got done at radiology. They were looking at my films now. Who has time to prepare for these things? Confer while the patient waits.

I waited.

Finally in he came, with Rubin and his nurse, Eugenie Johnson, right behind. We were a crowd in the little exam room. I got up to shake his hand with both of mine, not something I had planned, but this was the guy who could help me. He pulled back. Ken Offit is even shorter than I am, wiry, and with enough energy to power a small city, enough speed in the mouth to talk you into buying a half dozen bridges. I've lived through this scene over and over. If it seems to you I remember it too well, I can only say that this is the way it happened and that there aren't many more important, far-reaching conversations one has is a lifetime: a marriage proposal, how sex works, someone you love is dead, you have cancer. I can't think of the others right now.

"I know we're a little late," Offit said, "but the radiologists were actually interested in the case. Usually they treat us like garbage. But this they spent time on."

"Did the slides arrive from Knowles' lab?" I wanted him first to tell me I had succeeded in the job he had given me—submit all this stuff.

"Yeah, yeah. It's all good stuff. You should see what we get on some people. Didn't I tell you this would be a job? There are a few more tests we'd like to run. And some of Knowles' slides were illegible. Not everybody thinks he's the last word in lymphoma pathology. But, no, if you're thinking there's some question about the diagnosis . . . our pathologists are willing to sign off on it, which is good enough for me."

"I just thought . . . I didn't know maybe . . .

"Nah. It's lymphoma. Exactly what kind, we aren't one hundred percent sure of. But that shouldn't change anything right now. So what do we do? First put on a gown and we'll examine you." Eugenie handed me a gown, and Offit tore the curtain around the exam table. "Where's your wife?" he asked while I changed.

"She's working. She teaches upstate."

"Well, what's the story? Are you two together on this or are you on your own? Are you estranged?" Not the most delicate way to put the question, but since then I've understood how important.

"No. We're together. It's just that I've had so many doctors' appointments. She can't come to all of them. She wouldn't get anything done." But immediately I was sorry I hadn't seen this difference and told Jean to cut school and come.

"And this is just another doctor's appointment?"

"I don't know yet."

He whipped open the curtain. "Well, let's see what we have here. Sit up on the table." Offit and Rubin then examined me. They felt and poked around the neck and under the arms. What I was coming to understand as routine for lymphoma patients. "Lie down." They poked my groin and palpated my abdomen. "Sit up." I'd been through all this. Always nothing doing. Nothing cooking in Offit's words. They listened to my chest with stethoscopes. This part is important. The disease is in my lungs.

"No one has been able to hear anything, even with the X-ray . . ."

"Don't talk. He can't hear with you talking."

"But he's right. It sounds clear," said Rubin.

"Let me. Now Breathe. Again. Again. Again. You're right, can't hear anything. Even with that X-ray. Well, a picture's worth a thousand somethings. Put your clothes on." Close curtain.

In the little exam tent I heard them talking. Rubin had to go. It was five o'clock already. Nathan must be shitting a brick.

"Go." Offit said. "I'll give him the five options and try to get him up to Boston and I'll see you in the morning. Eugenie, can you hunt up a consent form for our study, and we'll give him that. Are you ready?"

Dressed again, I gingerly peeled back the curtain. Rubin was gone. Haven't seen him since.

"Sit down. So tell me, you went to another guy before you came here, right? What did he say?"

"That he couldn't find another case of mantle cell appearing in the lung only . . . "

"You don't need to worry about that right now. We've seen pulmonary lymphoma before. What did he say about treatment?"

"Either chlorambucil, which he said would not cure it . . . "

"He's right there."

"Or nine cycles of CHOP, which might."

"No way. CHOP will not cure this. Forget it. So listen, here are your choices, as I see it. Go to somebody else and you'll get another opinion. Don't take notes, listen to me. This will all be written up in a letter. OK. Five options. First, do nothing. You could probably go along like you are for a couple more years."

"Nothing? Isn't it time to treat this?"

"Right. I wouldn't have you as a patient with that decision. But listen, I have to give you these options. Second, chlorambucil. We already discussed that. Third, CVP. It's similar to CHOP. I don't recommend it. You couldn't do it here with me, but I have to tell you these things. CVP has side effects, hair loss, nausea, etc. You've heard all this. Like CHOP. And like CHOP, a dead end. Fourth, treatment with six cycles of fludarabine. It has virtually no side effects except for lowering your blood counts some, right, Eugenie?

"It is extremely tolerable," she said with a hopeful smile.

"There is a chance it might be the only treatment you will need," back to the main man.

"Really? That sounds great," I said. Yes. I knew there was a reason to come here. He's onto something better, more tolerable. Few side effects and gets the job done. This is it.

"I say a chance. It's theoretical. It could happen, nobody's tried it. I'm not sure exactly if you could do it here. But you would do it for a purpose. And that would be for a bone marrow transplant."

"What? Whoa." One moment I'm up. The next moment my heart sinks through my guts, and I almost loose it in my pants.

"We think that transplant is your only realistic hope for a cure. There are many advantages to going for it up front."

"What . . . what do you mean, up front?"

"You haven't been treated at all," said Eugenie. "Prepare for the transplant now, not later."

"Look, you could take any of these treatments and the disease will come back. When it does we have to treat you again before you can go to transplant. Why not transplant now while you are in relatively good health and can withstand the procedure?"

"I just. I mean, I had no idea. I didn't think it was . . . "

"What? Serious?" he asked.

"I thought you had to be a lot sicker before a transplant . . . "

"In the past, yes. That's what we want to study. Are you better off to transplant now, rather than later after the disease has come back?"

"Couldn't I take Fludara, whatever, and see and then decide?"

"No study will want you once you've been treated," Eugenie said.

"And I think you should go to Dana-Farber in Boston for the transplant." said Offit. We do it here, but in our study you could be randomized out, and I want to give you this extra edge. And Farber is better at this. We want to make you grandfather material. And you have family up there, right?

"Yes, I do." He had clearly given this a lot of thought. That's why he was so late. "What is randomized out?"

"The study has two groups," said Eugenie. "One gets the transplant and the other gets just radiation. You don't decide which you get. The computer decides."

"Did you find a consent form for him?"

"Right here." Eugenie handed me a sheaf of xeroxed pages.

"Take this home and read it," said Offit. "It tells you in there all about the computer. It also tells you in general what a bone marrow transplant is."

"Yee gods. What do I do about insurance?" I blurted.

"It's a medical necessity. They are supposed to cover it. This is your only realistic chance of a cure. But don't worry about the insurance now. First go to Dana-Farber. Get their opinion. Maybe they won't do it. Maybe they'll let you take fludarabine here and go to transplant there. You just don't want to do anything to ruin your chances for transplant.

"How do I? I mean, do I just call Dana-Farber . . . "

"No. I'll give you a doctor's number. But you have to go. They have to daven over you, you'll have to get them the films and slides, the works. In the meantime, I want you to have another bronchoscopy."

"I thought you had enough tissue for diagnosis."

"We do. That's not the issue. There are still some fancy tests we'd like to have. Set up an appointment with Dr. Stover. Maybe she won't want to do the bronch. But see her. There are two kinds of special patients, right, Eugenie?"

"The first are people we just like, cause we like 'em."

"And the other group are unusual cases," said Offit. "You made the second group already." Was I supposed to be proud? Was I supposed to work to get into the first group? Double my chances.

"Yeah, well, I guess . . . " I was pretty much of an idiot by now. These options and then transplant. And deep down I hoped maybe he'd come in and say the diagnosis was iffy. I had pneumonia after all.

"As cancers go, this one isn't the worst," said Offit. You have to decide if you are going for the first down or the touchdown. Talk it over with your family. Call tomorrow and the secretary will give you the number up there. Then let me know what they say. But get thee to Dana-Farber.

"I will. I'll call."

They both wished me luck. As soon as they were gone I was on the phone again. "Nathan, I'm on my way."

DAY FOUR

I've been crawling into the bed around two in the afternoon, completely worn to the bone. The bed, as much as I try to stay out of it, to sit in the chair for sanity and self-respect, or pace back and forth for exercise, the bed is a refuge, a reward for holding my head up for a few hours. By the time I pull back the sheet and ease under it, the place is home, the only place in the world I want to be, the only place that holds what I need most, finally where I belong. And soon I'm off to sleep and some remove.

But today as I lay my head on the pillow, even the bed was little comfort. I mumbled into the sheet—I don't know how much more of this I can take. If this is the way it is going to go on, if day after day I crawl with less and less energy into bed, if in the end I just don't get out of the bed, I just don't know . . . they're going to have to do something for me. Something else. I can't tell if they have me on a regular schedule of drugs, but every night the nurse asks if I want the Ativan. Should I say yes, no, maybe so? I say yes and sleep half the night. Should I ask Sandy for it during the day? Should I try without? I feel like absolute shit.

I woke up from my nap and lay motionless. Even after Jean came in, I kept my eyes shut. Let her sit, let her come gradually into the room. What did she need me grumbling at her? We'd been here before. In September, after seven cycles of the fludarabine, I had a surgical biopsy, a thoracoscopy, done by inserting a fiber-optic tube through the chest wall. The procedure saves the patient from having his chest ripped wide open, but the pathologists still get their tissue. Thoracoscopy does not take six weeks to recover from as does a full thoracotomy. But the day it was done, my side hurt like hell and I was pretty unpleasant to my wife, responding to her in angry grunts while to the doctors and nurses I was at least civil, even pleasant. And why shouldn't I be? The nurses brought me morphine, just what I needed after being stabbed three times in the chest.

I opened my eyes. We chatted, and slowly I came back into the world, as much as an isolation hospital room is a part of the world. Jean has been having a rough time of it. She is staying with her father only five minutes away. But he is post polio and has very limited time on his feet. It's enough for him to have Jean and Clare, and on weekends Nathan, staying with him. Jean does the extra shopping and cleaning. So between getting Clare to and from half-day day care, taking care of the three of them at home, and shoveling out the car to get herself here, she is pretty worn out. And now that the semester has begun, she is getting calls almost daily from her co-chair. Jean is the chair of the dance half of a drama/dance department. She tells me about the goings on at college. Now how could I care? But I am distracted to hear about the outside world, and she needs to talk to someone. She has all kinds of new headaches in the half year since she was made chair. The college is really being quite understanding about her absence, but it gnaws at her. Just as she was getting a grip on her new job, I have to go in for transplant.

She isn't getting the sympathy she deserves. Some friends have come through, like Susan who calls every week from Seattle and offers us both a telephone shoulder to cry on. Others have made themselves scarce. We started therapy right after the diagnosis and our therapist has been enormously supportive. Judy has brought forward the possibility that as awful as what I am going through is, the experience can be meaningful. For Jean it is mostly shit work. So she is distracted and helps distract me with her tales of who is in and who is on the outs in the college life she will return to sometime when I'm out of here and can take care of myself. Today she lets me close my eyes while she talks. But eventually she must go, not just to take care of our daughter, but because she must have time out of the hospital, and because, love her as I do, I must have time alone.

I remember leaving my mother in the hospital after a visit and going out to eat with my father. He eats on a schedule, three squares a day. We laugh when he says, "Eat now; you'll be hungry later." In his twenties he had an ulcer that put him on a schedule he hasn't broken. It doesn't matter what he eats, as long as the timing is right. But a couple of times we went from the hospital to very nice restaurants, places that my parents would go to only for special occasions. At that time it was just a night out and away from the hospital.

So I imagine Jean just leaving at eight or ten in the evening and taking herself out to eat and being on her own in a restaurant or bar. Nobody knows what she's going through, and that's just fine with her for the moment. But halfway through her second drink, it isn't fine. She wants everyone to know that bone marrow transplants, wonderful as they are to give hope where there was little ten years ago, suck out loud. But she tells me that she's too tired to take herself out, as my father had as a kind of consolation. She goes home to her father's apartment, makes sure Clare is sleeping all right, and sits up with a drink in front of late night TV for an hour. Sometimes we talk on the phone late at night.

Most of the time I find TV too hard to watch, though now and then when all else fails, there is always TV. Larry tells me that some patients keep the TV on all the time, even when they sleep, and wake up and complain if a nurse turns the tube off. TV is a companion who knows nothing and asks less. A hole in the wall through which you see the world outside, not a very clear or accurate picture, but a very insistent, color one. I can't focus too well on the screen. I can't focus too well on anything. Sleep today is only a slight respite. I'm woozy and shaky on my feet. There is so much I want to tell you. The months of treatment. I have to tell you about my mother, and how I've lived with somebody's cancer most of my life. You'll want to know what I do when I'm not dealing with all this, which I almost cannot remember, and about my family, and what I'm reading. I want to tell you about the acupuncturist, the healer, and more about therapy. How am I going to get all this said? I can barely focus my eyes, let alone my pen. Oh please, please, just let me go back to sleep. If only I can rest, I'll feel better. But I am resting. I'm in bed barely moving. How much more rest can I ask for?

DAY FIVE

Another lousy day. Not enough energy to do yoga. I can get up to go to the bathroom, but that's about it. I am too tired to read. The page is a blur. Figuring I should have a choice, I brought a pile of books, but who can read when you can't focus? I'm looking at *Young Men and Fire* by Norman Maclean. I loved his *A River Runs Through It*, but this is something else again. The book is an account of a troop of young smoke jumpers caught in a firestorm in a place called Mann Gulch, western Montana. The event took place three months after I was born, right across the street from where I now sit trying to read the same paragraph over and over. There's probably something to this coincidence, but I haven't the energy to figure it out. Since Maclean died before he edited the book, it's filled with repetition. But I can't tell whether Maclean is repeating himself, or if, in my haze, I'm rereading passages I read last night or two days ago. I can't tell if I'm repeating myself now.

Why on earth have I brought into the transplant room a book about young men being burned to death? Why not Woody Allen? Why not fall asleep with the TV on? Play comedies on the VCR all day? What's the matter with me? I'm flying blind here. Last spring I dutifully rented a few comedy tapes to take the laugh cure. In the middle of *A Fish Called Wanda* I had to pee. Standing in the bathroom, I called out loud—Oh my god, I have cancer. Remembering so abruptly was a nasty surprise. I trust Maclean. He's taking me somewhere. He keeps his eye on death. By keeping an eye on death, I avoid nasty surprises. I have had it with nasty surprises.

Late this afternoon, I felt warm. I keep the thermostat high; people remark on how warm it is in here. I usually don't like hot rooms, but I have no energy to spare to heat my body. Like other ordinary hospital tools, the thermometer lives in the room so as not to bring bugs in from outside. Why wait for the nurse? I took my own temp. 101. This means business. I called the desk. "I have a fever now." Spotter to base. We have a fire in the Man's Gulch.

In another minute, Gail came in and went to work on me. She felt my forehead, and popped in the thermometer. Can't trust the patient. Even before it beeped, she went ahead drawing blood. Not just a CBC, but tubes for lord knows how many blood cultures, including one from each lumen of both catheters, and from a vein in my arm. She took a throat culture, a swab around my mouth, each ear, up my nose. "Go pee into this cup and save everything that comes out of you for cultures." The drill was on. Find the source of the infection and get the right antibiotic to pounce on it. This is how bone marrow transplants have improved over the years, new antibiotics and antiemetics to make the whole deal more survivable. Does it cure more people?—We don't know Mr. Seder, that, what we are studying. Glad to have you aboard.

As Gail left with her tray of blood tubes, I asked what would happen next. "Do we wait for the results?"

"Oh no. We start you on antibiotics right away. Then when the results come in they adjust or switch or whatever. Have you been taking the Bactrim?"

"Trying, but I keep gagging and throwing it up." Besides acyclovir to prevent herpes, they have me on Bactrim to prevent PCP. But the Bactrim are horse pills, and I'm not doing too well swallowing jello.

I heaved a sigh. OK, ready for the next step? It isn't enough to feel sick, now I really am. Pretty soon a tech showed up, and while

I stood in the doorway, shot a portable chest X-ray from the hallway. Back to bed. Take temp again. Send puke and shit to the lab. Then Gail reappeared with some meds. "They want you on mezlocilin and gentamicin. The mez is every six and the gent every four hours. We'll be in and out of here changing bags a lot."

She hooked up the pump and the mez started running in. Coupled with the transfusions I am now getting, there will be little room in my busy schedule for young men on fire. Vey is mere. Wake me when it's over.

DAY SIX

Mez and gent, and platelets and red cells, and G-csf. G is a hormone that stimulates the production of white cells. It was developed at Sloan-Kettering and given to Sloan's patients free of charge. Otherwise it's about a hundred and twenty-five dollars a shot, and when I was taking it outpatient, I gave myself a shot every day for eight days. I'm not right now supposed to be worrying about money. It will drive you crazy, says Bonnie, the social worker here. One thing at a time. Bad for the immune system to worry, right? Money can kill me, right? I won't be the first.

But G is good stuff, said Dr. Offit when he started me on it. The first week I came back to his clinic with a white count of seventeen thousand. "Am I giving myself the shots right?" I asked.

"Either that," he said, "Or you've come down with a sudden case of leukemia." Fun guy. He described himself as a Harvard-trained attack dog. Grrrr. Rip out the heart of those malignant cells. Throw the dog a bone marrow.

But G only works as long as you have stem cells to make blood, and right now I have zilch. Sandy has started a chart on the wall recording my daily blood counts. On days when I get transfusions there are two counts, a before and an after. I have less than one hundred white cells per unit. Normal is above 4000. They want me up to 1000 before they will open my door.

This is the bad time. With no white cells to fight off infection, I am vulnerable to every little bug. All the stuff your body fights off without your knowing, I might get. It's like having a temporary case of AIDS. Temporary sounds as if I'm sure that the bone marrow will engraft. No one has said it might not. But they did say that without evidence of disease in the marrow, a donor transplant would be too risky. Which I took to mean using my own marrow wasn't so risky. Temporary, as if I'm better off than someone with permanent immune disease. As if I have a lesser or cleaner disease. As if I have more right to hope. What I have is bad enough. And the chart Sandy put up is pathetic. Less than 100 really means uncountably small.

But the fever has not gone up. I'm stewing, but no worse. The dentist came. They send a dental resident every few days because I can't use a real tooth brush for fear of causing the gums to bleed, which, with no platelets, could be a big deal. But at the same time they have to make sure the teeth are getting clean enough so I don't wind up with infected gums. Sandy told me, as if I'm her little kid, "Don't stick your fingers in your mouth. If you get something caught in your teeth, we call the dentist and they take it out with floss. Very carefully." I can't even floss myself. Of course it's hard to get jello caught in your teeth.

And the dentist keeps an eye on the mucositis. My mouth on its own fills up with glop; because, I'm told, of the effects of the radiation on the salivary glands. So added to my bathroom trip is a trip to the sink to spit out the muck. One nurse told me to swish baking soda, but that does nothing. Then came Kathy who suggested an old-time remedy, Alkalol. Of course she can't get the stuff in house, so she bought me some on her way to work. Does the trick, at a dollar a bottle.

And Kathy is a dear, dear woman. Straight from the hip, a lifetime of caring written all over her face. A no-nonsense, sophisticated lady who has the sense not to be constantly bubbling. There are times the nurse just can't make things better. It plain sucks. Kathy doesn't use that language. She says—rough going, you hang in there. Jean loves Kathy. She told me how Kathy pulled her aside and told her that this week would be the worst, the bad time.

They check my vitals more frequently. How many times can one person have his blood pressure taken? It's low. It's always been low. Now it's lower. If I have no blood counts, how can I have blood pressure? They give me transfusions and I guess I have plasma. Where does it come from? Maybe I'll ask Rob tomorrow.

Rob Soiffer is the attending on service this month. He visits me every afternoon. We go over the counts, how I'm doing, if I need anything. The intern has examined me at seven, and the fellow comes in later in the morning. Rob doesn't have much physical business to attend to; get his eyes on the patient, listen to my voice, find out if anything needs adjustment. Rounds must be held in the morning, when Jared Goleb, the transplant fellow, comes in. At first I didn't think they did rounds, but one morning, looking out my peep hole, I saw the whole gang in the hall in conference: Rob, Adam the intern, Jared, Sandy, other nurses, the infectious disease doctors, the dental resident, the pharmacist. A big crowd. But only Jared actually came into the room. They want to minimize my exposure to outside bugs.

Jared is a good guy, soft-spoken, always gives time for any question, seems to enjoy explaining and doesn't mind if I ask the same thing I asked yesterday. But he looks like one of us. The guy is skinny enough to be a patient. His pants will fall down any moment. Maybe he does have some condition, and is not just skinny. After all, isn't one's own health problem a good entree into medicine? Not for me, thank you, but for someone.

Right now none of them has anything new to say to me, but—Hang in there. I'm hanging.

DAY SEVEN

I must have something pumping around my veins. After all, I'm still thinking. I'm still talking to you. You hear me, don't you? What is in the veins? Water? Plasma with nothing but borrowed cells from the IV bag? You can keep red cells for a couple of weeks. Platelets last a few days. Lini says I should have decent walking around counts within a month of getting out of the hospital. That doesn't sound as bad as the year I read about.

Let me tell you about Lini Pandite, the Farber doctor who brought me here. I love her. She is gracious and caring and thoughtful. She is Sri Lankan and has the most beautiful deep brown eyes. There are few eyes I have looked into with such intimacy. The rest of her is pretty good looking too. My wife says she's afraid I'll run off with Lini, which in my current condition would be suicide. Jean thinks it would be pretty nasty in any condition.

Lini gives me her time in the exam room and on the phone. In the period before we made a definite decision to go with the transplant, we were on the phone a lot. I had had the seven cycles of fludarabine, then the biopsy, which showed lymphoma still, and then at Lini's insistence three cycles of CHOP chemotherapy. Then I had another CT to find out if the CHOP had any effect on the lungs. If then there were no signs of disease, Lini said the transplant would have the best shot at the cancer. If the CT still showed signs of disease, but as we knew already much reduced, then I would be considered in "minimal disease state" and still a candidate for transplant. I thought the choice was mine.

Then came the December night she told me on the phone that

she needed to take my case to a committee, and my tears on the Broadway island as my anger built at the chance that this committee might send me back to start, and my little epiphany in traffic—Yes, Lini, I want it.

When she called a few days later to tell me that everything was a go, she said the sweetest thing. She had been kept awake at night worrying about me. I knew I wasn't sleeping well. But I was the one with the cancer and having to make this decision. She was the doctor. Why was she awake? If I weren't in minimal disease state, the transplant would be a waste. She quoted one line from the committee, "Lini, what are you waiting for?" Maybe she had internalized my doubts.

Even still, doubts lingered. I thought they were completely reasonable. I mean, look at me now. In her office I asked Lini what she would do if this were her. "You know the disease, the procedure, my case better than I do." She hedged, at least that's what I thought at first.

"Look, that's a hard thing to answer, Bob. I do not know. Yes, I know all these things, but the disease is not inside my body but in yours."

I wanted an answer in no uncertain terms. But for the nine hundredth time I was told there is no one way to get through this, no one else is precisely you, you are alone with the beast that can kill you. To go for the jugular or nibble away at the scales is finally an expression of who you are.

Today I say that I wouldn't have trusted an unhesitating response from Lini—Yes, absolutely. Go for it! She wouldn't say such a thing, and that's why I love her. But at the moment, she made my life only more complicated and difficult.

Anyway, here I am. On this service the attending physicians

rotate inpatient coverage. Lini is not on this month, but she stops by for a visit now and then. A few days ago, she came and said I looked pretty good, considering. But the mask doesn't hide those lovely, slightly sad, brown eyes. Jean asked her a few questions; we chatted and joked—We'll have you out of here in no time, hah hah.

As soon as she was out the door, I threw up. So much for getting out in no time.

DAY EIGHT

I'm woozy and shaky and queazy, but I'm not throwing up and the fever is going down. Something isn't right about my IV pump, and the thing starts to buzz a warning every once in a while. Apparently the antibiotic keeps getting stuck in the tube, and I have to call Dave at the desk, and he has to send in the nurse to fix it. A royal pain when I'm dropping off to sleep, which can happen at any moment. The nurse has to suit up to come in and flick a few air bubbles out of the hose and reset the pump.

Larry finally showed me how to turn off the beeper so I wouldn't have to listen to the thing while he washed, gloved, gowned, and masked just to spend fifteen seconds tapping the hose. But after five minutes the thing starts buzzing again. Larry takes two or three pushes of the button to get in here. He'd be quicker I know in an emergency, but this is just a nuisance. "Mr. Seder's thingee is going off again." Larry also told me why the problem persists: "Cost. They want us to try this new hose which is a couple of bucks cheaper. I say chuck the whole rig out the window."

"Go for it."

"But then where would you be? Wouldn't you miss my company? Now please keep this quiet long enough for me to have my lunch."

"It's two o'clock in the morning."

"Yeah, we used to call it the graveyard shift, but that didn't sound too good around here. Nighty night."

People come to visit. Cousins Judy and Henry have been a real help this past year, listening to my accounts of doctor visits, lab reports, general unhappiness, and terror. They are both therapists and have a low threshold for any unkindness shown by a doctor or anyone else on staff. They can speak all the med talk with the best of them, but it was Judy who gave me back the phrase "It plain sucks." They look uncomfortable in masks and gloves and ill-fitting paper gowns. I wish visiting me weren't the cause of their awkwardness, but if I were to say this, Judy—I love her for this—would have my head off.

When Richard, another cousin, visits, he doesn't look awkward for a minute. He's a pathologist and enters the room pushing the door open with his back, his gloved hands raised and ready for action. We should all have a doctor in the family to interpret, to ask questions we lay folk can't begin to form, to ally fears, and express awe that comes from both compassion and knowledge. Richard's done this and more. We've spent hours on the phone rehashing and questioning details of the diagnosis and treatment plans. He helped in the search for second opinions and had the slides looked at by a colleague. He even called and talked to Dr. Offit, who now refers to him as the other Doctor Seder. He apologizes for not staying longer, but really his timing is perfect; get eyeball to eyeball for a few minutes, that's what counts.

I am glad they come. I want to see people. But in ten minutes I have to close my eyes. I never had any idea what nurses meant when they said—Don't stay long, it will tire him out. What the hell, I'm just lying in bed, how tired can that make me? Very. Smiling takes energy.

I can't bring myself to ask people to go or to wait in the lounge for a while. Will they come back? It's snowing again. They had to shovel to get here. It's cold outside and very warm in here.

How can I send them out into it?

My father visits. After my mother died, he remarried, and now he and his wife live in a retirement community, a managed living arrangement.

"How are you?"

"OK."

"Good. You look OK."

People say this to me. What the hell do they mean? I don't look OK. I wish my cousin Michael would visit. He'd say, "Vey is mere, Seder. You look like death warmed over. Come, I'll take you for a walk outside in the blizzard, give you some color." But Michael lives in California and my sister lives in Israel.

My father means well. He says to me, "I don't know what to say to cheer you up," as if the necessary thing to do is to be more cheery. And since he has decided, with good reason, that really there is little cheerful he can say, he says little. What must it feel like to see his son looking so awful, going through this horrendous procedure, facing a life-threatening illness? It must be painful. This isn't the way things are supposed to be. My father is seventy-eight. The wrong guy is in the bed. I asked him once how this felt. He told me it didn't matter what he felt, I was only to get better. But here's the thing, Dad, my knowing you are hurting might help me feel less alone. But no, not cheery.

So instead he talks about his will. He is doing this thing for taxes and that thing for my sister on the kibbutz and something else for the grandchildren and giving some away. I will be the executor of his will. A lawyer cousin I barely know will be co-executor. I will have to make sure my sister and her children get their share. At first I simply couldn't believe my ears. I am in the bed, in an isolation room, in the cancer hospital. He's the visitor. He walks out of here. What is going on?

I'm tired. I don't talk much. Well, Bob, look, this is how he deals: either in total denial or the threat of death triggers—Write the will, deal with death as with everything else, think ahead, research, plan, finalize. But yeesh. I wonder if moving to this retirement place—where the only people he sees are old, where someone is always dying, where everything looks snazzy, but the place is still the end of the line—was such a good idea after all. The idea, he always said, was not to be, in your old age, a burden to your children. And right now I have to say this looks like a pretty smart move to this weak, bald, sallow child who wants no more burden than sleep.

Can I take on his pain? Not today. But I need to know I mean enough in their world, that my cancer and my living in this room cause the people I love some pain. Doesn't have to be what I feel. But hurt lets me know I'm not alone. We are all holding it in. I am dying for a breath. A free, easy, deep breath. A sigh, a shout.

In the period after I got sick and before the diagnosis came down, the period when we still thought I might have some lingering complicated pneumonia, I went many times to the radiology lab for chest X-rays. I learned to recognize what the doctors meant by the infiltrates on the films. Once, riding the elevator back to Dr. O'Sullivan's office, I pulled out the films to check them. The image looked different to me. My heart leapt into my throat. Holy shit, I'm getting better. It's come at last. Look, look. Better. My whole body was zinging alive. How much had I been holding in going from one day, one appointment, one test, to the next? I always had hope, but that's a different feeling from seeing success.

Mary O'Sullivan explained to me that all X-rays look a little different. They call it technique, how the film is shot and developed. Just as you can develop a snapshot fuzzy or sharp. This image was just sharper than the others. The infiltrates were still there.

"Look at the bones," she said. "Presumably they don't change from one week to the next. The bones are the same." Burst my bubble. Pretty pictures are not a cure.

My father would like to cheer me up. I will cheer, when the X-ray changes. If it doesn't, I'll have to find some other way to get at the lightness I felt the day I misread the film.

The other day, Denise came to visit. She's been a friend for I don't know how many years. She obeyed the dressing rules, but didn't even pretend to stay off the patient's bed. She plunked down next to me and held my hands. Her rings made funny bumps in the gloves. We didn't say much, just held onto each other for nowhere near long enough. I could have fallen asleep on this visitor. Before she left, we hugged at the door, and, on her way to the elevator, she peaked in the window with her mask off. She didn't look too cheerful. Seeing her was the high point of my day. But she wondered if that hug would be the last.

DAY NINE

Do I think more people will visit more often? It snows like crazy every other day, and no one can get around. They have their lives to live, business to attend to. Nathan needs Jean on a school visit. This one has a meeting, that one has school. I'm making excuses. It's lonely in this room. Here's the question: Would I visit? If you go in next year, or whenever it is I'm allowed into a hospital again for civilian purposes, I'll come visit.

I sent a letter to family and friends a month or so ago when it looked certain that I would be coming in. I didn't want to hear later—Oh, I didn't know. Better give them the gory details and let them decide what they want to do. Some people were on the phone right away. "I had no idea how serious. What can I do? Where do I go to give blood?" Some I haven't heard from still.

I tried to keep it from being a weepy letter, to stick to the facts and treat our need as another fact in the case. I brought the leftover copies in with me, heaven knows why. "We are going to need help," I wrote. "It isn't so easy for us to ask, independent types that we are. But we are bang up against an enormous need, navigating at night through a storm at sea, the leading lights into safe harbor a memory lost in the fog."

A little much, that metaphor, but I won't be sailing these waters again. I was gearing myself up. Maybe the people I haven't heard from were offended by the frankness. I was long past the point of privacy, of—Don't talk about it and maybe it will go away, and people treat you better if they don't know the details of your sickness. Maybe you lose their respect, as if by giving it your all you are caving to the illness and not saving something for the rest of the world, for them. Tell me again what I need this respect for? Especially if I don't make it?

I'm daydreaming about the island on Grand Lake in northern Maine, the base for the wilderness canoe trips I went on as a kid. This summer, if I live, it will be thirty years since I was last there. Sometimes when I can't sleep I take myself back across ten miles of lake and come ashore at this place that was a wonder to a suburban kid, a wild place where I was protected but free to lie in the lap of the lake, at peace with water and sky, the loons and the bugs, sunburn, nasty lazy campers, sore muscles from paddling all day, and constant hunger. In a jiff I would trade constant hunger for constant nausea. A few years ago I got myself back on the camp mailing list and learned that the director was ailing. I wrote him my feelings about the place and the time I had spent paddling his wooden canoes through the wilds of Maine. I meant the letter as praise for the wonderful idea he had brought into the world and sustained with great care for almost thirty years. He took the letter as reminiscence. He died the same summer I got sick. At least I got that letter off in time, turned that stone.

If you come in here next year, I will visit you. It can be lonely in here, but you will have great company. If you must be isolated in a room like this one, know you are the most interesting person out of all of us. Nobody who's suffered in this bed or will suffer in it, will do it the way you do. No one deserves the chance more, and no one is better company. But the guy in the bed right now, I sometimes find a crashing bore. Nighty night.

DAY TEN

I'm exhausted from anemia, from the relentless day after day–ness. I don't know if I can go on with this story. And I've left out all kinds of stuff: mortality and morbidity rates, toxicity to organs, the recovery time, the people I've talked to who've had transplants, how attractive the young women in dark blue coats at Memorial are, the hours on the telephone. I'm too tired today to talk. But did I tell you Offit said that very first day, "We want to make you grandfather material"? Nobody before or since has said anything like that. And here I still am.

Nothing doing on the counts. No fever. I'll be back tomorrow.

DAY ELEVEN

It's happened. When the blood report came back this morning, the white count had budged. It isn't much, about one hundred. They need one thousand to open my door and about four is the low end of normal. But today's count is not nothing. G-mcsf works better, Jared says, on stem cells than G-csf, which works better once the marrow has engrafted. A stem cell makes three kinds of cells, which in turn make the three kinds of blood cells, white, red, and platelets. G-m stimulates growth, but it can't do anything without stem cells, or early stem cells. That the white count moved means some marrow has engrafted. Did I just say this? I'm on the way, moving at last. I'm eating soft foods, and there's a sign of bone marrow again. On the move.

Sandy was happy. She uncorked the magic marker and boldly wrote 100 at the bottom of the graph, but not at zero. The other counts went down. Yesterday I had a platelet transfusion which had bumped them up to fifty-seven thousand. Today they are down to thirty-eight thousand. When I came in, the count was a hundred fifty thousand and change. The hematocrit is down as well. Lini says the platelets lag behind the other counts and not to worry. Does that explain the red count's bouncing around? Too soon to tell anything.

Now that the counts have started to move, we have other business to take care of. "Well you aren't staying here forever," Sandy said. "It's time you cared for your own Hickman. If you leave with the catheter, you'll have to do this at home." And she proceeded to teach me. She's a good teacher, but the process, for a first month nursing student like me, is not easy. First clean the work area, the little tray table. This much I can do fine. But everything else is supposed to be done in a sterile field, and I wasted a couple of dressing-tray kits getting the hang of it. It makes me nervous. I could be giving myself bugs. But hell, I can handle it, I got a hundred little white blood cells running around inside.

(You can skip all this dressing kit stuff if you want to, but talking it through helps me remember what I have to do.)

Next I peel the clear film bandage off my chest. First they teach not to touch the thing, then how to yank it off. Then I open the plastic bag that holds the sterile tray. So far, so good. Now things get touchy. The tray is wrapped in a sheet of waffle paper folded so two flaps appear on the top. I am supposed to pull the outsides of these flaps open to expose the contents of the tray. Now everything inside is available but sterile, and I mustn't touch it until I have the gloves on. The gloves sit on top. With two fingers, I pick up a glove on its inside, the side that will touch my nonsterile skin, and slip my other hand inside as far as it will go. Sandy can get all five fingers into the right holes in one fell swoop. Me, I'm doing great if I get one finger into a hole. "Not to worry," she says. Now the gloved hand is sterile, and I have to pick up the second glove with my one sterile finger hooked into the rolled cuff of glove number two so that the sterile finger touches only the sterile outside of the other glove. When both hands are covered, then I can rearrange the fingers because sterile glove can now touch sterile glove.

I'm breathing hard and sweating, and only now am I ready to get down to business. There are two packages of swabs in the kit. The alcohol swabs are supposed to be on top. I pick up the foil pack and rip off the top. Drop the foil top back on the tray. Reaching for the trash can, I'm too likely to contaminate the sterile field accidentally. Now pull out a swab, and starting at the point where the catheter enters the chest, swab the skin in a widening circle. Never back up, because you might carry a bug back onto the cleaned area from the dirty. Three swabs in the pack, use them all the same way. Then open the Betadine swabs and do the same. While I wait for the brown stuff to dry, I keep my gloved hands raised and inert above the sterile field. You've seen the TV doctors do it. Now rip open the little ointment package and ooze a drop out onto the site. Place the sterile pad over the site and peal the back off the clear plastic bandage and slap that sucker over the whole mess. Breathe. Wrap the junk in the once sterile waffle paper and toss it away. All there is to it. Should have been a doc. Oh shit, I forgot something, but I can't think of it. Never go from unsterile to sterile. Or from sterile to unsterile. Do not put the swab package down on the table and pick it up again. The mask. I'm supposed to wear a mask the whole time. Good thing I'm not leaving tomorrow.

It's simple living in a clean room when somebody else does the cleaning. Now Sandy wants me to do it. She promises to watch when I repeat in three days, and Adam will check the site every morning. "Once you get out of here," Sandy sang her mock-serious tune, "there'll be no Sandy or Adam to check on you. Next time I'll show you how to flush the line." She meant the inside of it with needles and heparin-filled syringes. I can wait. Until then . . .

DAY TWELVE

Even with no fever, they still have me on the mez and gent and will keep me on them until I get a white count of a thousand and a poly count of about half that. Polys are a part of the white blood, important in fighting infection. Polys are good. Even a thousand whites won't open the door if I'm low on polys. Today I ain't got no polys. Try me again tomorrow.

With all this changing of antibiotic bottles and transfusion bags, and the damn tubing that keeps getting stuck and making the pump alarm sound, I have people coming and going at all hours. I don't even bother in the middle of the night to talk over the intercom. I just hold down the bottom and let my IV pump do the squawking. Larry was just in to fix the tube yet again.

"You know, it costs them more for me to fix this—do you mind if I say—fucking thing? This is your room, after all."

"Be my guest."

"I am your guest. The visiting nurse in yellow cape. Every time I fix the fucking thing, they lose me on the floor just so I can tap a few air bubbles out of the . . . thing, and they can't really save more than fifty cents a shot. Now look around this place. How far is fifty cents going to get you?"

"Not even across the hall."

"How long have you been in here?"

"Nineteen days."

"Well for you, my friend, it will probably cost fifty thousand dollars to cross this hall. Ven ve let you. So hurry up already and get some blood counts, so I don't have to tend to this . . . foolish thing, and I can get some sleep on my shifts."

"But other patients must have the same tubes."

"No, my friend, you are it. The only one on this med. Solo. It's all a scheme on your part to get extra attention. You've rigged this up to make that infernal noise every five (fucking) minutes. And it prances nursie hot off the cot."

"Your smiling face does the heart good."

"Smiling face? How would you know? Under this mask is a grimace, my friend. Actually, I wrote in my report that this tubing experiment is a total waste, except for the amusement it gives Mr. Seder. So of course they keep the tubing."

"You didn't."

"I have to write something. It's too boring everyday to write, he eats, he sleeps, he shits, he watches Mary Tyler Moore reruns."

"I have never in my life watched Mary Tyler Moore and I intend to keep it that way."

"At the rate you're going . . . Sorry. Bad taste. I owe you one. For your amusement we keep zee tubes. But apres vous, le garbage."

"I think it should be la garbage."

"Le garbage, la garbage; when you go, it goes. So get some counts, will ya."

"I'm working on it as hard as I can."

"You can say that again. My job is a piece of cake compared to what you do. Now the lying in bed all day part I could take, but all this throwing up and shitting in hats, and fevers, you can take it. Which you seem to be doing pretty well. As well as anybody I've seen around here. And I've seen a few. What was on tonight?" We were following the winter Olympics.

"Tonya Von Buelo arrived in Lillihammer."

"Big news day."

"She got off the plane, kissed the tarmac, and said, 'What's the Norwegian for sledge hammer?'"

"Crow bar. Crow bar. You have to keep your weapons straight. You would stink at Clue."

"I was good at Clue."

"Give your marrow time to grow back. I had Chris spike it with the contents of that little black envelope."

The squawk box interrupted. "Larry, please state your position." A euphemism for—Where the hell are you?

"I am tubing—or is it de-tubing—Mr. Seder."

"We need you to assist in fourteen."—Move your ass.

"I'm on my way," Larry shouted toward the mic at the head of the bed. "You've had your Ativan already, so I'll just hit you over the head with my crowbar so you can get back to sleep."

DAY THIRTEEN

Yes. White count two hundred. And fifty polys. On the move. Yesterday I asked Rob Soiffer if the counts usually take this long to come back. No. I am in the slower half of patients. I picture what I can remember of the corridor outside my room and imagine most of the people in those rooms with more counts than I have. But today more movement. So, OK, go with what you got. Sandy warned me not to expect a steady climb. "Some days it goes up. Some days it goes down. But you will see the general trend will be up."

And Bonnie told me not to focus too much attention on each day's progress but look at a larger picture. "Today's count may be barely more than yesterday's. But a week ago you had nothing." Right, Bonnie, now that you put it that way.

Snow again tonight. The sulfur vapor street lights turn it yellow as it falls. When I get right up to the window I can look down on the roof of the lower floors. The roof is strewn with old car tires, fast disappearing under the snow. What are these tires doing there? No car could have been stranded up here even in the highest tide. Were the tires leftover from the construction? And no one paid enough attention to take them down? The tires are sad remnants of something or other, left over scrap, used up carcasses of once useful parts. Us. The ruined marrow we've left behind. I will have to leave something of myself inside the Dana-Farber Cancer Institute. You give a piece of your heart. Doesn't mean it won't grow back bigger, but the left-behind part is still behind. If I have to leave a part of me, it may as well be my used snow tires.

The window sticks out from the side of the building in a shallow bay. And just now, very close to the glass, I can see into the bay of the room next door. There's a warm light on in there and a plant on the table. Plant. We aren't allowed plants and flowers, they carry bugs. Maybe she has a fake plant in there. As if a hospital room weren't complete without one, real or fake. Why she? The plant? The ribbon in the plant? The snow tire? I'm thinking of my mother's many hospitalizations.

I was six when she was diagnosed, and she went in every year for at least twelve years after that. To us kids, her trips seemed normal. Cancer was normal in our house. She didn't say cancer until I was into my twenties. She said tumor. She said disease. She said axilla not underarm. Did she say breast? She brought presents from the hospital gift shop. She didn't swim. She was proud of her doctors. She would come home from a test and say that this was all very interesting and would be educational if it weren't her body they were testing. I made her breakfast while she recuperated and sometimes supper. When I was a teenager she went back to school to get her MSW. She would not be stopped. For years she bounced back from each episode when nodes were removed. Until the disease became general. Then bouncing wasn't so easy, but she continued to work.

So after the first shock of my diagnosis wore off, I was surprised by the feeling that the inevitable had finally happened. Without being conscious of it before, I saw that I couldn't possibly not have cancer. I had always told myself that I was relatively healthy. I kept a balanced diet, ate little meat, was a moderate drinker, former smoker, vitamin taker, health-conscious guy who, like everyone else, did what I could to avoid cancer. But once I was faced with it, I saw I wasn't like everyone else. Whether cancer is in the genes, it is in the family and in the psyche. (How do I propose not passing this on to my own kid? First I accept that I may not be able to. Genes are genes, and the kids will be hurt and scarred by my illness. But I will use the word: cancer. How can they hope they avoid it without its name. I will try to teach hygiene. I will try and talk about it. I haven't been too good at this. I will do everything to stay alive; yes, as a model to them, but first for me.)

This feeling of inevitability took weeks to articulate. And now I have another feeling. I have been waiting thirty something years for the other shoe to drop. A year ago it did. Now, instead of being terrified or paralyzed, I became energized. Here it was at last. It showed its ugly face and now I have a chance to smack it hard. Cancer is a fat, ugly, hairy rat that sat down in the middle of our family, and even if we can't heave it back out wherever it came from, we can elbow it out of the way, make it sit still in the corner and shut up.

Right in these few blocks my mother spent so much of her life. Something of her fighting spirit is here, watching.

The light next door goes out. The lady in there is going to try to go to sleep.

If they had been doing bone marrow transplants for breast cancer sixteen years ago, I know my mother would have gone for it. As it was she tried a number of experiments. If I learned anything from her disease, I learned that cancer is survivable. Look, she survived year after year, treatment after treatment. The people who would have me think always positive thoughts would approve, but a permanent positive attitude would have had a negative side for my mother. She would have had trouble truly convincing the young man I was then, just coming into my own and having seen her survive year in and year out, that this bone marrow transplant business was the ultimate seriousness.

She wouldn't have that trouble today.

DAY FOURTEEN

Hippidy hoppidy. Look at this, counts doubled again overnight. Four hundred whites and a hundred polys. We are on the road and moving in the right direction. Just the numbers make the blood pump faster, put a little more air in the top of my chest. Yes, yes, I'm going to make it. Yes, Elizabeth, we are beating this sucker. I remember this feeling of the lightness of success: in an elevator looking at my chest films, convinced that they were clearing, and later as I got off the table after a repeat gallium scan. The heart just jumped up into my throat.

Last July, after the first six cycles of chemotherapy, Offit ordered another CT and a gallium scan of the whole body. When Mary O'Sullivan sent me for the gallium, six months before, the lungs had lit up like bright charcoal on the scan. Offit wanted to compare and see how effective the chemo had been.

For a gallium scan, a patient gets an injection of a radioactive isotope, comes back a couple of days later, and lies under a camera that collects the emitted radiation remaining in the body. Positive areas will take up the gallium, normal won't. The CT can only see the surface of the stuff; it cannot distinguish tumor from scar. The gallium can indicate cellular activity; within limits it can tell what is going on inside what the CT shows.

Did the chemo make a difference? Neil Spector, my first doctor at Dana-Farber, said that if the CT turned out to be abnormal, but the gallium normal, then we could assume that the CT showed scar tissue, not disease, because between the two galliums I had taken chemotherapy. Offit wasn't so ready to put his faith in the gallium. Richard Seder explained the problem. A reactive process will also cause the gallium to light up. In other words, if anybody bothered to do a gallium scan of a patient with pneumonia, the lung would also light up.

Going into the test, I was back in the I-don't-know-what-to-want mode. With all the disease in the lungs, nobody really expected the CT to be clear, but the choices went like this: CT and gallium abnormal would mean active disease. CT and gallium both normal would mean remission. A split decision would mean:

"You have gotten benefit from the chemo," said Richard, "a partial remission at least."

"Good news," said Neil, "a good sign of remission."

"Surgery," said Offit. "Tissue is the gold standard. It's the only way we know what we are looking at."

Gulp. I thought we were done with surgery talk. I buried Offit's comment. Take the scan and get the results.

Like everything else at Memorial Sloan-Kettering, the gallium scan was easier, quicker, more assuredly performed. Plus the TV monitor, instead of sitting far across the room, was placed so I could easily watch the image of my body being drawn over the half hour I lay still. Every once in a while, the tech repositioned the camera, and I got to wiggle. When it was all over, I stood in my exam johnny and stared at the twirling orange figure of what I looked like to this machine. The tech flipped through a few different views for me. To me, the left lung looked as if it had cleared up completely.

"But the other lung. What's this big blob at the base of my right lung?"

"That's not the lung. That's the liver."

Holy shit. Metastasis. I have liver, cancer. I'm going to die. When it got to my mother's liver, she said, "You don't live with liver cancer. You only have one liver. They can't take it out. This is it."

"This is normal," said the tech.

"Huh?" What was the guy saying while I was fixing to die?

"The liver normally takes up the gallium. Where was your disease?"

I snapped to keen attention. He said, where was your disease. "In the lungs."

"Oh. Well you should get a good report from this."

All right, all right, all right. Good report. I paid my dues. Here it is, pay back time. Good report. Remission. This means just what Neil said it means. Remission. Remission. Rest. No more chemo for a while. Give me some time away from all this. Get me out of this hospital. Get me away from sickness and cancer. Get me into the mountains. This means I can have at least what's left of the summer. This means . . .

"Surgery," said Offit. "You are cruising to an open lung biopsy. It is the only way we can tell. We can't leave you without knowing. The biopsy is your ticket to the transplant."

How much bouncing can one heart take?

To the rescue came the pulmonary department. Early on I had Mary O'Sullivan; now I had Diane Stover and her fellow, Gail Schattner. From the second bronchoscopy through the months of chemotherapy, they insisted on following me along with the other docs. While Offit and Neil davened over the causes and the course of treatment, Drs. Stover and Schattner looked at the effects. While the oncologists were worrying about the difference between the gallium and the CT, the pulmonologists looked very carefully at the CT and saw, "wonderful improvement. Really very encouraging. This is amazing."

And Dr. Stover said I wouldn't need the open lung biopsy. "I'm almost sure the surgeon will be able to get tissue from a video assisted thoracoscopy. This is a much less invasive procedure, and it has a much quicker recovery period. We'll send you to the best."

I liked this team long before they saved me the trauma of the open lung procedure. Because of Dr. Stover's many patients and other responsibilities as head of the department, I spent more time in the exam room with Gail. She began almost every visit formally and seriously, as if part of her fellowship was practicing her doctor face. Maybe she kept it up with other patients, but with me it didn't last but a couple of minutes, before she broke out in smiles. Gail is warm and funny and gives generously. She does not avoid, as some docs do, going eyeball to eyeball. This is serious intimate stuff, you deserve direct contact with your doc.

In our first visit, I showed her the chronology that had impressed Offit's fellow. But Gail said, "This is good, but let's just talk." I love her. She has an unstudied instinct for healing that she can only have brought with her to med school. When I told her that my breathing seemed easier after I started taking vitamin E, she leaned across the table and, practically in a whisper, said, "It's good that you feel that way, but you know doctors don't really believe in vitamins."

Her voice has just the right mix of assurance, concern, and wonder. She let me know that she had to think about my situation, that she couldn't answer off the top of her head. The energy of that thought and her letting me know about it is healing. And she has unusual hands. Gail's hands are normally cold. Very cold. I stiffened when she laid a hand on my shoulder while she listened with the stethoscope. She said, "I know. I'm sorry. Some of my patients are old ladies, and they almost jump off the table. I should remember to warm them up." Maybe. Or maybe the cold and the zing it gives you, along with her soft voice, is something like the laying on of hands. Cold hands, warm heart.

I wouldn't mention this zing—it might embarrass Gail, but I love her for that too—were it not that last fall I started acupuncture treatment and experienced a similar, if more focused, zing from the needles. For months I had taken the chemo, relieved finally to have a treatment program and not still be hunting for causes. I had simplified my diet and drank more water and less coffee and alcohol. I already practiced a bit of yoga, but I tried, in a relaxed way, to add meditation. I didn't want to leave out the chance that an alternative approach might do some good at the point I was approaching the decision on the transplant.

A friend had given me the name of her acupuncturist, and I kept his number among all the doctors, appointments, blood slips, report numbers, in my illness notebook. I am always going to the book for one thing or another, sometimes just to see if there is something I've forgotten. I had forgotten Bob Abramson. I didn't know exactly what acupuncture would do for me, but was suddenly antsy about not trying. How could it hurt?

Bob Abramson is not Chinese. He's a few years older than I am, but only looks it because his hair has gone entirely white. He was a dentist, then became an MD, then an acupuncturist. Lots of school for this guy. But what a relief to talk about the lymphoma and the treatment so far with an alternative medicine guy who, as an MD, understands more than I am saying. I really didn't want someone who was about to bad-mouth Western medicine and my doctors. I had already been through this with a homeopath type, who thought she was doing me a favor by pointing out how arrogant and mistaken my doctors' approach was. The mind shut down. But Bob is entirely sympathetic, serious but always ready to follow any ironic twist. We laugh a lot in his office. Whatever he can do with his needles, his voice alone is healing.

"So what do you think acupuncture can do for you?"

"I'm new to this so I don't really know. But I'm facing this surgery. So first I'd like to be as strong as I can be to get through it and recover. If the biopsy result is negative, I'd like to strengthen my immune system and keep it that way. If the result is positive and I have to face more chemotherapy and then the transplant, I want to do it in as good shape with as healthy an immune system as possible." I had expected his question and had studied this answer.

"That's a tall order, but get undressed and up on the table and we'll see."

He felt the pulses in my wrists. Don't ask me how acupuncture works. I only know in the very vaguest way about the pulses, energies, meridians, points, and the five elements. Bob said he couldn't explain. It would take him five years. He held my hand as he took the pulse, and I told him he has the smoothest hands.

"Well you know, this isn't exactly construction work I do here." If laughter is curative, give Bob Abramson another degree. I've tried my bit to keep him healthy too.

With his eyes closed, he felt the pulses in both wrists, wrote some notes, and then treated me with needles. I tried to relax on the table and breathe slowly and meditatively. This I can tell you about acupuncture: against infection, he swabs the skin with alcohol first, the needles are tiny, and they don't hurt. The only surprise was when he pulled the first needle out with great force. I got a zing from it, a little like Gail's hands.

He said I should come back again. We shook hands, and I floated out of his office.

I don't know what Bob did, but I felt wonderful. I drifted out onto Broadway and just couldn't bring myself to get onto a bus. Jean was picking up Nathan at school a few blocks away. Maybe they stayed after in the playground. I'll glide on up and see.

"My God, what happened to you?" Jean said when she saw me. "You are positively glowing. Look at him," she said to the mother of one of Nathan's friends. "You look great."

I saw Bob a couple more times before the biopsy report came back positive and I started CHOP chemotherapy. I was very disappointed when Offit insisted that, while my counts were lowered by CHOP, I stay away from acupuncture needles. Bob even talked to him on the phone, but we decided I had come this distance with Offit, I would be a fool not to stick to the program.

While everyone else was busy keeping up my hopes for a negative biopsy, Offit's hunch was that I still had active disease and he cautioned me to get ready for more chemo. I have to give his hunches weight; he's more often right. But it hurt to give up acupuncture even temporarily. It was something I was doing for myself. I did not like having it taken away.

My therapist I did have, and we talked through all this stuff—I was about to say, talked to death—until it was almost manageable. The laying on of hands, meeting the healer eyeball to eyeball, the give and take of medicine, couldn't have got this far without it.

But even a few pleasant memories get me all tuckered out. Just making words is a drain. Until tomorrow . . .

DAY FIFTEEN

What's this? What is going on? Four hundred whites. I had four hundred yesterday. Everyday since they started to come, the counts have gone up. Now this. Polys though are up to one forty-five so that's something. This waiting. You can have it. OK, come on, come on. Sandy draws the blood. A couple of hours later she comes back with the results. If there is a chance I'll have low platelets—today was OK at thirty-one—she won't let me do the yoga until after the report or after a transfusion. The way they have been dropping, tomorrow she is going to make me wait. Sandy says, "The counts bounce around. We've seen this before. Not to worry."

"But Rob said this was slow."

"That may be. But we've seen much slower, believe me. This happens. You're doing fine."

"This is fine?"

"Well, what did you expect?"

I was talking about acupuncture and therapy, things besides the medicine I did to deal with this thing. Jean and I went together to therapy within a week of diagnosis. Judy Nenner has been terrific. She's listened, talked, and cried with us. She helps bring meaning to this experience. It matters not only that I go through the transplant and survive it, it matters how.

After the thoracoscopy, we waited ten days for the biopsy results, an unconscionable amount of time, and Judy was the most angry about it. "How dare they make somebody wait day after day. Do they have no idea how important this is?" No question I was anxious, and towards the end was calling Offit's secretary everyday. But I kept thinking, the results must at least be ambiguous, questionable, which is a step up from certainly malignant. In the end, the delay came only from the pathologist's interest in the case; he did a complete review, films and all. As Offit said the first day, "Usually they treat us like garbage, but this interested them."

Of course Judy and everyone else were wishing for a negative finding. She pressed me for seeming ambivalent. "How can you not want them to find nothing?" Did she suspect I harbored a death wish? That wasn't it.

"They've told me the disease is incurrable by conventional therapies. Even if they can't find it, which would be great news, that doesn't mean it isn't there. It just means they can't find it, and are willing to stop treatment until it pops up where they can find it. I dearly want to stop treatment, but if they find it now, that means that I go on to transplant, and transplant may mean the route to a sooner cure. I don't know what to want."

"What an awful place to be at." Her questioning got me to put into words, probably for the first time, that this horrendous procedure I'm living through right now, is, for all its messiness, my best chance at life. Through months of therapy we had avoided talk of transplant. We let it loom on the horizon and left it there. Now it was upon us.

I told Judy how I completely astounded myself by changing focus as Offit was giving me the news. Before he opened his mouth, I was saying to myself—It's going to be good, I know he'll say remission. Halfway through the conversation, I was asking, "When do we start CHOP. The sooner the better as far as I'm concerned." No time today for yesterday's dream. Oh but did I cry over today's loss.

I had never been to a shrink before. Did I think I had had enough of them with my mother a psychiatric social worker and cousins doctors and shrinks? I was proud to have taken care of myself, whatever that meant. (Was I foolish, a part-time lighting designer, part-time writer making little dent in the world as either?) But cancer has a way of focusing the mind, to say the least. I don't have to do this on my own. This is what help was invented for. My turn at therapy had come.

We were very lucky to have hit it off with Judy, though finding her was not luck. Our good friend and neighbor, Mary Soyer, herself a social worker, sent us. With or without Judy I would have wound up in this room. But the how would have been different. I arrived, if not in one piece, then at least aware; I made a choice—an awful one, but mine. Judy was there, not to make it, but to help tease out the details and the feelings that allowed me first to frame the choice, then to realize that I did have to decide, then finally to decide, and after that to give me confidence to hold on to the doubts, and to change my mind if I had to. "You don't have to go through with this just because you said you would. You can back out right up until they put the needle in your arm. Even there, you still have a choice." By needle she meant that first bag of chemo. By then I was resolved, but she had me know I was in the driver's seat.

I am very wary of anybody who tells you you have to do this or do that to fight cancer. I get angry when people say: you absolutely must seek second third fourth fifth opinions (though I did wind up with at least five); you must give up meat (with low blood counts I started to eat meat); you must be aggressive and noisy to get good care (I try to be personable, but persistent); you must take laugh therapy (I dearly hate the jolt back to cancer reality as soon as the VCR. switches to rewind); you must keep a positive frame of mind (this is fucking cancer, my life is threatened, if you don't call this negative you have your head wedged in a very dark spot); you must confront your doctor; you must relax; you must get out more; you must take alternative therapy. No, it is harder than all this. You must decide for yourself how to face this dread. Even passivity is a choice. But, do what you want, I cannot see surviving cancer treatment without psychotherapy.

I am still the most interesting person I know. (The same goes for you.) Worse things can happen than having to spend a month in a room with me.

"Yeah," said Judy, "you could turn out to be a schmuck."

Laugh therapy.

DAY SIXTEEN

Tired to the bone. No yoga. Platelets down to fifteen. Crit dropping. Whites down to three hundred from four the last two days. Polys down to eighty-five. What is going on? I don't want to talk. I'm taking a nap. Leave me alone.

DAY SEVENTEEN

Long, tiring day. Platelet and red cell transfusions. But the white count is back up to four hundred and the polys to ninety-six. I was hoping for more. I was hoping to jog out of here. And I don't jog. Jared can't tell me why the counts are bouncing around and won't take off. Rob Soiffer can't tell me. Lini can't tell me. Why don't I stop asking. Not for nothing are we called patient.

But the red transfusion has given me a little more energy and I'm awake and at the window again. The view at night is not so very different from daytime. Those tires on the roof. They don't have anything to do with snow. It's the heat. They keep the roof from buckling in the summer. By summer I'll be lying on the beach, completely shaded of course and chilled by the cool sea breeze, these heavy snows will be long forgotten; someone else will be suffering in this room.

Binney Street is well lighted and I can see down onto a small section of Longwood. All the hospitals around me are ablaze. Between Children's Hospital and Brigham is a wide swath of air straight out to the east and over the harbor. At night especially, I can see airplanes approaching Logan Airport. The nighttime view of Boston from the air I've seen many times. Did a patient standing in this window look up one night and see the blinking lights of my plane, and was I looking down at him and having no idea what I was seeing? I have an idea now.

Most of the windows in Children's Hospital are either dark or show a faint glow. Right at my level is a window with a purple Barney dinosaur pasted to it. Behind that window is a little kid, old enough to talk, but probably not to read. In the corner of the room is a reading lamp. I imagine the child asleep. But slumped in a chair in the corner is an anxious parent trying to read or write or somehow pass the worried night, to be there if the child should wake and need mommy or daddy. I imagine a while ago they ate supper with the youngster (or maybe the kid is on chemo, and the parents don't want to insult her by eating what she can't eat right in front of her). Poor kid barely knows what is happening to her. After supper, the parents have a quiet but intense argument. Tonight is the father's turn to stay. Last night he went home early. One of them has to get some sleep. But tonight his wife didn't want to go.

But you have to get out of here for a few hours. Get some rest. I'll stay. I have plenty of work.

Nah, I won't sleep any better at home, she says. I spend the time on the road. I get home and call you, and I can't sleep for worrying.

Have a drink.

I can't have a drink. What if I have to come right back?

But I'll be here.

But if something happens.

I'll be here.

I want to be here too. Will you call me? If she wakes up and asks for me, call me?

You have to get some rest.

I'd rather stay than let you maybe decide not to call me.

If you don't go, you will be a basket case by morning. You don't need that. I don't need it, and Meagan doesn't need it. She needs you alert. Not dead to the world.

I'll try. But I might come back.

Go.

And reluctantly she takes the elevator to the parking garage, pays the reduced rate, and drives home to Millis or Malden or Mattapan. What a wonderful simple thing to do: ride an elevator, drive a car alone at night with the window rolled down and the radio on. When's my turn?

Now he rests in the glow over there. Or maybe he can't rest. I conjure all this, but really, for the life of me, I can't imagine what I would do if it were one of my kids and not me in here. At least I can suffer and take what has to be taken. I know the kids are affected, but it is very different to visit a parent in the hospital than it is to live in here yourself. I've played both roles now. I say a little blessing for the child across the way and for her parents. Have strength. Come through. Get well. Bear what has to be borne and live this out. All hope to you. And I say a little blessing for my own kids: Daddy says take a good look around my room; with luck you won't be seeing the likes of this for a long time.

Later I see the man at the window with the phone to his ear. His wife can't sleep. He can't read. I can't read so I go on with their story.

How is she?

She's asleep. She's been asleep since you left.

Is that good? She hasn't been sleeping through the night. Not while I'm there.

What can I say? You want me to wake her up to see if she's alive? Should I ask her if she has to puke?

No, I'm just saying she keeps waking and not sleeping like this. Has she been like this with you?

No, but please. Thank heaven for a few hours sleep. You do the same, will you?

The nursing assistant comes into my room and turns the light on. She has to check the hat in the toilet. Everything that goes into me is measured. Everything that comes out is measured. Wouldn't want anything to get lost inside.

Jeez there's a guy over there in a johnny. He's looking right into our room.

A guy? Over where?

In the hospital across the street. He's standing right in the window, I can see where the light just went on. He's standing right there watching. He's not moving. How long's he been standing there?

What are you talking about? What difference does it make, somebody's standing in a window?

Nothing. But I feel like he's watching Meagan. What hospital is that?

Across Binney?

Yeah, right there.

The cancer hospital.

You think the guy is a bone marrow transplant?

How do I know? Is Meagan asleep still?

Yeah.

Then why don't you draw the curtains and go to sleep. Forget the neighbors, and think of your own.

The nursing assistant leaves without a word. I turn off the light after her.

Light's gone off over there. Can't see that guy anymore.

Good. Go to sleep.

Me too. I must be doing a little better if I'm worrying about the people across the way, not that I know the first thing about them.

DAY EIGHTEEN

On the move again. Whites up to six hundred and polys one eighty. Highest for both. Yes, on the go again. Jared says they are thinking about changing the white blood stimulating hormone from G-mcsf to G-csf. He says when there are even some small counts this shift might give them an extra boost. Why, they don't really know, but they've seen it happen. He didn't order it today. He and Rob will look at the counts tomorrow morning and decide. He said to call him if I have any more questions. OK. When can I go home?

Jean's sister-in-law visited. She has been an enormous help to Jean, especially taking Clare now and then in the afternoons. When Jean flew to New York and back one day to take Nathan to a school visit, Gerry took care of Clare. For the last year or so she has called more often than before, and last week she sent me a note.

She said she finds my stoicism inspiring. Am I a stoic? At heart? Do you think so? To you I blab everything, more than you'd care to know probably. I don't strike you as a silent sufferer, do I? Silent? That the blab doesn't land everywhere, doesn't mean I don't blab. What is a stoic? Wait, let me look it up. "Unmoved by joy, grief, or pain." Is that what I am? "Submits without complaint to unavoidable necessity." That part pertains—maybe. But it took months of chemotherapy, the surgery, the many opinions, and psychotherapy before I would submit; or rather, before I put aside the complaint and made of the decision an act of affirmation, not submission. Is that a bit of the stoic's philosophy at work? Or is it a practical response to a devastating reality? (I'll look up pragmatism tomorrow.) Or is it a trick of the mind to pretend to want what you have little control over?

Maybe Gerry sees something here I don't. Or maybe she wants more from me than I can give. What? Maybe she wants me to let her be the healer. Or maybe she wants to hear the scream from deep inside this fiery furnace. I'm not Shadrack; I would never lead the way. And Meshach follows his brother blindly, does what his doctor tells him to. So I'm Abednego, doubting, turning back to the world left behind, like Orpheus, but in the end, cannot live without his brothers and takes the plunge. Maybe this whole effort of day by day conversation is an answer to Gerry's blunt question: What's it like? This is it, Gerry.

The healer. Judy Nenner pointed me at another stone she thought I'd better turn. A friend of hers is a healer. What healer means I still can't say, even after I visited Sandy a couple of times. But she has a touch. As I lay on her carpet, she went into something like a trance. She said she went inside. With me in a meditative state she got our "auras" in communication and brought healing powers to bear on the sick parts of me. I have no training or judgment about what she did. I know that I would not rely only on this sort of thing without medicine. Could spiritual healing, the laying on of hands, the moving of energies, imaging, meditation have curative value? I know tons have been written on the subject, and I have barely read a pound. What harm does it do unless it leads you not to take your medicine? Perhaps it makes you more open to the healing potential of the medicine. Perhaps it makes the side effects more bearable if you can visualize the medicine at work. People argue about this, and I have no answer. But Sandy taught me a few meditation techniques to try while I'm here, and sometimes I do them. When I have no energy to talk or read or even to open my eyes, I can still "run the energies" as she taught me. If it gives me nothing else, it allows me to participate in my healing.

So today I did the yoga in the morning, meditated as I went down for my two o'clock nap, and rode the stationary bike for twenty minutes listening to the radio.

When I lived in Cambridge I would listen to WBUR through the day and night if I was working at home. They used to have a wonderful mix of personalities, opinion, and offbeat radio humor and drama. Now the station has become completely bland and homogenized. True, if I am sick to my stomach and listen to them, who can tell where the sickness is coming from? But they had a good thing going and they blew it. What they did to BUR is like what they did to Boston's West End—gutted it.

Shush. I'm an old elephant come home to die and can't find the watering hole under the parking lot. I tell you, with awe at the poetry of it, that from this window you can see the place I was born. But that building is no longer the Boston Lying-in Hospital. It's now a records warehouse for Brigham and Women's. Don't get me started. Progress has carelessly ripped down and cemented over the sites of our memories, but it has given us G-csf, the Visitel, video thoracoscopy, mez and gent. It keeps us alive long enough for Sandy to work her magic by laying on a hand, or Larry the voodoo of laughter. It takes a whole culture to invent a bone marrow transplant. Hooray for that, but it makes me awfully tired.

DAY NINETEEN

Counts are mixed. Whites up to seven hundred, but polys down to one sixty-eight. Bumpy ride. Jared said that the counts are about where they have to be to open the door. But they will try today changing to G-csf and wait till tomorrow. I don't know what to think. You never know anymore. Tomorrow they may go down again. I'll have to be patient now that generally we are moving in the right direction.

Yesterday I mentioned Visitel. What the hell is that you asked? When Offit had to tell me that the thoracoscopy biopsy was positive, he also recommended that I see a shrink at Memorial. Another shrink? He must be crazy, but I took her name anyway. The more I thought about it, the more I warmed to the idea of seeing a feelings doctor who also knew the medicine, someone who actually worked the transplant floor. I met several times with Mary Jane Massie and we talked easily and well. Judy had me trained. Now I had a specific, time-limited problem: should I go for transplant and if so how to prepare.

In a way, Mary Jane, the psychiatrist, dealt more with what seemed to me social work and practical issues, while Judy, the CSW, worked on the underlying feelings. Dr. Massie arranged for the loan of a Visitel, a video telephone that sends snapshots over the telephone lines. The transplant unit at Memorial has a grant to use these things for families from out of town, to help the patient keep in touch. Dr. Massie wants the people at Farber to get in on the grant. The thing is pretty primitive, someday we'll be able to send real time moving pictures. With this you have to pose in front of the thing, stop your phone conversation for a few seconds while the machine sends the person on the other end a picture of you with the phone in your ear staring at the Visitel.

We left one Visitel with Nathan in New York and the other sits by my bed. Nathan sends pictures of Mary and Kayla and Jerry and I send pictures of me—bald, beardless, and fifteen pounds lighter. It's only black and white so they can't see how pale yellow I look. The thing is a conversation stopper, but keeps Nathan on the line longer than he would be otherwise.

"OK Dad, you sound better. Wait right there, I'll get Mary and Jerry, they want to send a picture."

"I'm not going anywhere." And he runs next door to get the crowd. Nathan is living in both apartments at once.

"OK Dad, we're ready to send." The machine buzzes and whines, and after a few seconds a not quite sharp snapshot of the four of them staring down at my desk at home wipes down the screen. They're smiling. I guess Nathan is OK. He's known Mary and Kayla all his life, their apartment is almost another home for him. Have I got this far into this deal without talking about Jerry?

Jerry is a biochemist. His lab is at Sloan-Kettering. He is, in his words, a high mucha there. He helped get a second opinion there. He visited me in the hospital there. At every important juncture he has asked pointed questions. He has to know what we know and then says—Get another opinion, or—Believe me, this is safe, they do it every day, or—Look you have to know this is not a death sentence. We go to him frequently for advice. We've always known that if there were some serious disagreement between the doctors or some major screw up, Jerry would be there to help resolve it And he pulls no punches. I look sick, he doesn't tell me I look pretty good, he says, "You look like shit, what are they doing for you?" To see his enormous smile next to Nathan's warms my heart.

The beeper on my pump still goes off but we don't pay much attention. I'm tired, but a good riding-the-bike tired. Tomorrow is another day. We'll see then if the counts come up at all. I don't want to say hope for the door open. It will happen when it happens. I'm not staying here the rest of my days. When Nathan was little and we worried about toilet training, a friend with long experience said—Look at it this way, no way the kid is getting to be twelve years old and still in diapers. Relax. Soon is all I know. I do hope that at least the weather clears up, and Jean doesn't have to shovel out the car and can sleep later. Here comes Larry with my Ativan. In a few moments I'll be asleep. You sleep too. Doesn't listening to all this make you tired?

DAY TWENTY

This is how it happened. Yesterday they switched to G-csf in hopes of giving the white count a boost. But the platelets and crit have been falling for three days. I'm cruising toward transfusions today or tomorrow. So after Sandy drew the blood, she said, "No exercise until the counts come back."

"OK, whatever, I'm not going anywhere." I paced window to door, door to window. The counts are taking longer than predicted to come back. I stuck my face in the little window a few times, and finally, Dave, the guy at the desk, held up his copy of the *Globe* and asked if I wanted the paper.

"Aren't you reading it?" I shouted through the closed door.

"Too busy now. Give it back later." And he shoved it into the pass-through. I sat down and looked at his paper. There was a follow-up on Jackie Kennedy Onassis's lymphoma. Jean told me they had debated whether to tell me about it. As if I would feel threatened knowing there was more lymphoma in the world? That it was all around me, and there was no escaping it? As if I had no more room for someone else having as much difficulty myself? Either I'm totally out of it and denying like crazy or they just don't get it. Why should her disease be more of a threat to me? She has a high-grade lymphoma, which may be related, but the course of the disease is totally different. And when famous people get sick, the disease gets more attention. Could that hurt me?

I turned the pages half reading, crime, corruption, and cancer. I still can't focus my eyes for very long. I'm only three quarters of the way through *Young Men and Fire*. I slammed the paper down onto the bed. I paced. I peered out the little window as if looking for them would bring the counts. Dave waved. I went back to his paper. Finish it before he wants it back. Another page. What difference does it make whether I read his paper or not. Where's Sandy with my counts?

I pace. The sports page. How about those Knicks? Finally, Sandy stuck her head in the pass-through.

"Are my counts back yet? Can I do my exercises?"

"Not yet. Wait a minute, I'll go check." Jeez. Why does she bother me if she doesn't have any information. And what's the matter with her face? Why isn't she wearing a mask? Well she wouldn't have to in the pass-through; the air from this room blows only one way.

But the next thing I knew, Sandy had whipped open the door and stood in the opening, no mask, no gloves, no gown. "This is it my friend. Your door is now open. You are free. The next door that opens for you will be the main entrance to the Farber."

I was stunned. I couldn't move.

"C'mon," she waved me out.

I stood up, walked slowly to the open door, and leaned against the door jam. Sandy wasn't alone in the hallway. A small crowd was waiting for me: Jared and Rob, Kathy and Gail, Dave, and other nurses and assistants whom I only recognized from my window. They started to applaud. I almost fell over. I inched my way over the threshold and leaned against the wall, now on the outside, if only just. They kept clapping. My knees were about to buckle. I couldn't see through the tears. Sandy strapped a mask over my nose and mouth.

"New rules. Now you have to wear the mask and we don't. But only in the corridor, in your room no mask." Then she gave me a big hug. Me and her baby. She looked so healthy and glowing without the mask. Then hugs all around. Kathy had a tear in her eye as she handed me a ribboned bottle of sparkling cider. A year I would wait for champagne. She knew all this intimate stuff about me, but I had never seen her nose before. It was bigger than I had imagined. Gail, who took care of me when the fever hit, gave me a big hug, a rub on the back. And there were congratulations all around. And even after they stopped clapping, and I had slumped back on the wall for support, they still didn't go back to work.

"I lobbied to open the door yesterday," said Jared, "but Rob said no. His call."

"We didn't want to take any unnecessary chances with you," said Rob, and gave me a quick hug. Nurses make better huggers than doctors, except for Lini.

"You're free. Why don't you go for a walk?" Sandy said.

"I will. I will. Let me get my legs." I felt as if I had just come ashore after weeks at sea. "You can't see it, but my face hurts from grinning. And this mask is all wet." Finally, as the staff did start back to work, Sandy took my arm. "Come. I'll take you for a walk."

Arm in arm she showed me the mundane but until now invisible sights of the floor: the conference room, the little kitchen, the pharmacy, storage, the nurse's back room, the two waiting rooms; Jean must know these pretty well by now. Too bad she isn't here yet. God, I have to call her.

Nearing the end of our loop, Sandy stopped in front of the elevator. "The next time you get into this elevator will be on your trip out of here. We keep you long enough to make sure that your exposure to the outside doesn't throw you back. Usually about three days. While you are out of your room you must wear a mask. Hospitals are pretty toxic places. You might be asked to move to another room if we need the transplant bed. Your cooked food diet will stay the same for a month. When people come to visit you they should wear a mask in your room if they have any runny nose or anything. But otherwise you have the run of the floor."

We wound up in the quiet lounge, the one with the little meditation chapel, just a few doors from my room. "I'm going to leave you now. I have to go back to work. Have a nice time."

I walked around the room a couple of times. The full-length windows looked out on a bright crisp February morning. Tired, I dragged a rocking chair over to a window and sat. From here I could see Beacon Hill and Back Bay. What a small, compact, confusing, and pretty city Boston is. And to me so homey. What a clear day. I can almost smell the crisp air. Fenway Park is over there. The old Sears building. Yee gods, Wheelock Theater where Jean and I first met. Have to call. And right in front of me, at my feet behind a new parking garage, was the Beth Israel Hospital where my mother had been a patient.

Then it all welled up inside and boiled over. I started to cry and cry, for her, for all her suffering and early death, for our disease, for my sister and her daughter hospitalized for depression, for my cousin Judy's double hip replacement, for my grandmother's sudden dementia at ninety-three, for all this suffering and pain. The worst was over, and I overflowed. Joy, relief, grief, all mixed up. I cried, but the bright winter sky smiled.

I feel as if I've hiked up Mt. Washington in winter, and from here I can see forever, the long uphill struggle, the icy route down the other side. But for the moment I have survived, and in that chair I cried long fat tears of relief.

Finally, I took myself for another walk around the floor—weak and slow, but joyously out of that room. In the other lounge I could see into Brookline Village and the top floor of Jack's building, where Jean and Clare had spent the past month. No picnic that.

I walked back to the room, a new little swing in my arms, a

wee bounce in my step. I sat on the bed, pulled off the mask, and called Jean. We cried over the phone. She knew the door was about to be opened. Jared had told her it might have been yesterday. She would leave Clare with Jack and come right over.

I called my father. At first he didn't quite understand. What on the face of it would be the big deal about opening a door? But when he pictured it, he said, "I don't know why, but I'm crying."

"Me too. I just cried my eyes out." And started again.

"Didn't I tell you everything was going to be OK," he said. Whoa, everything OK? That's going a little far. Always the son. Of course if he had said, Thank god, I was afraid you weren't going to make it, I would have contradicted him there too. Some stuff it takes more than radiation to root out.

I called Dr. Offit at Memorial and for once his secretary put me right through. He was effusive as I had never heard. "Congratulations. You aced it. You were due for one. Call me when you get back. And keep it up."

Jean was very tired but beaming. She looked so beautiful without that mask on. We made a plan for her to bring Clare this evening. She left after lunch.

I called Judy Nenner. "What exactly does door open mean?"

"It means the worst is over."

She heaved an enormous sigh. "Mazel tov. My fingers are relaxed."

"Fingers?"

"Can I uncross them? A little?"

I could feel a nap coming on, but kept my eyes open until Nathan would be home from school.

"Go turn on the Visitel," I told him in my most commanding father's voice.

"What for?" another contrary son.

"I have to show you something." He got the machine ready. "Here comes the picture." I lifted the thing up and pointed it at the open door and pushed the button to send.

"What's that?" Nathan couldn't tell on his end what the hell was going on. Why send a picture of the wall?

"Look carefully."

"Oh my god. Dad. Your door is open. That's wonderful. When are you coming home?"

"They'll keep me here for a few days and then I'll have to stay in Brookline for a week, anyway. "

"Oh. Well I'm coming this weekend, anyway. Is mom there?"

"She'll be back later with Clare. Will you tell Mary that the door is open?"

"Sure. Is that all?"

"No."

"I love you."

"I love you too. Bye."

DAY TWENTY-ONE

Yesterday the white count reached one thousand with polys of 410. Today, Sandy has changed the way she records the counts. For regular people, the decimal point is moved over three places so that a count of one thousand is reported as 1.0. Today I have a white count of 1.2 and polys of 510. So why don't I feel even better?

I'm hung over from the emotions of yesterday. Clare came in the evening. The guard downstairs insisted that a two-year-old wear a mask in the building. To make it more comfortable for her, Jean agreed to wear a mask too and cut one very small to fit on Clare's Barney doll. I was never so happy to see this puffy purple creature. Sandy, pregnant with her own little one, couldn't take her eyes off Clare. I wore a mask too, and we played in my room. We found stuff for her to monkey around with, some cups, a few blood tubes, and specimen jars, the soft foam tooth sticks. She was impressed to find her own drawings on my walls. What a bittersweetness to have this young soul playing with medical junk right in my room and walking the halls with us. That she is here means that I am on my way out of here and home. That she has to come at all, that she hasn't seen me these weeks and that I look so different now, bald again, paler and thinner than ever, what effect could this have? What kind of memories are we building in her? We can't ignore the disease or hide or pretend that everything is OK, but we don't want her to feel desperate. Will she remember anything? Will she remember the Barney doll with the mask? Is this more than a two-year-old can cope with? Would having no idea where Daddy is be worse? Should we have brought her in the first day, before any treatment, so she could keep some picture of Daddy's room in her mind?

Don't know. We have done what we have done. We will try to listen to her. We model sickness, we model how to deal with sickness. We love her throughout and hope love boosts her immunity to despair, fear, and numbness. For her I would not be sick, but I can't do that. For her I will do my best to stay alive. What else can I do?

Last summer, a friend of my in-laws sought me out because she had recently been diagnosed with breast cancer and wanted to compare how we dealt with our young kids. She decided she would tell the child only that she had a tumor. The word cancer she said would be too scary. I understand why she said this; my mother did the same when I was little. But I chose to use the word cancer because that is what I have and because I didn't want my kids to hear from somebody else—even in the most well-intentioned tones—How's your daddy's cancer? And because when years later my mother did use the word, I felt that I had been lead on, gypped. And she lost out; if she had cancer all those years and survived as if it had been "only tumors," then how threatening could it be? When her disease (I don't always choose the word cancer, do I?) did become general, my sister and I were unprepared for the seriousness. But this young woman had made up her mind how to deal, as had I. Instead of trying to convince each other of the value or terror of the word, we appreciated the camaraderie of the afflicted and left each other with a hug and good luck.

But why have I felt mopey, low, and edgy all day? I'm afraid of the outside and of what happens next. I'm afraid of being on my own. Of being a phone call, not a buzzer, away from the doctor. Whatever Jean has done to get by this month, I'm about to change all that. The dietician came by today with a list of restrictions:

cooked food only, no fresh fruit, no salad, no leftovers, no take-out food (which they may have been living on) no sharing of portions, separate dishes, separate small serving boxes, jars, and cans. Don't go near the stove. Shower everyday and wash the shower before I get in. Wash the toilet before and after, but I can't do this washing myself. No crowds, no restaurants, limit visitors, none with colds. No alcohol for a year. No intercourse until the platelets are fifty thousand, then use condoms. The list goes on. How are we going to manage? I have zero energy. What will it be like when I have to walk up stairs just to get to Jack's kitchen?

The hospital is really not as safe as it seems. I may be close to help, but I'm also swimming in a soup of hospital loving bugs, some of them potential killers. But I will miss the attendant cleaning the john and room, and changing the bed. How will I be able to do anything? I am so tired.

The walk around the floor has quickly become just exercise, not mountain climbing, but trudging through sand. They have stopped the antibiotics, I'm not pushing an IV pole. Without much ado, I've become a fixture around the halls. On the other side of the floor, I ran into the nurse who gave me the first bag of chemo and never came back. When I told her I had had only one fever and mucositis, she said: "Oh, you sailed through it." As if I should have nothing to complain about—Shut up you, we have some really sick people on this floor. And if I had had serious life-threatening complications, she would have made them out to be the fault of my body; that I go on living is due to the heroism of her staff. Walk away, walk away, walk away. I have not an ounce of energy to spare this woman. She will have to live out the next forty years of her self-tortured existence without the benefit of my blessing. Good luck, lady. Oh. That is a kind of blessing. Walk on.

No, I'm too tired to walk. I'm dead tired. I'm crawling back to bed. I wish I felt better. I wish I could get back some of yesterday's optimism and buzz. But it's all dulled, fatigued, and scared away. I have to go on, I'm scared to go on. I have to get out of this place, I'm scared to be anywhere else.

DAY TWENTY-TWO

Tomorrow is the day. I'm getting nervous and excited. I walked the floor before breakfast. There are very sick people here. We even found the friend of a friend from New York having a transplant for leukemia. We talked through his window. "How you doing?"

"Fine. I just took my Ativan." I never thought to ask for Ativan except at night.

I had transfusions yesterday, and have a little more zip in me today. The white count continues to climb, 1.3 with 637 polys. I don't ask what would happen if I stopped G-csf, but surely this would drop, and without red-cell transfusions, enormous fatigue would put me straight to bed. But red cells and platelets can be handled outpatient once the white count is high enough to look like an immune system.

Everything I don't need for overnight I'm giving Jean to take home. The notebook computer I never touched, the radio I can do without for a night, the sweat suit I never put on because the hospital will not wash it and I couldn't give Jean one more chore. Yeesh, she looks tired. I can see her harboring every ounce, every spec, of energy. We walk the floor and collapse onto my bed.

She went to a few sessions of a family support group. Everybody's situation is different, but of the spouses from out of town, Jean is the only one with a kid here. She got to chatting with a woman from Michigan whose husband is just coming out of a serious bout of pneumonia; Kathy worried he might not pull through. Their kids are at home with grandparents, and she spends all her days with Kevin. She misses her kids like crazy and says she can't do much more than hold Kevin's hand. But Jean, with Clare in tow going back and forth to the bus station on weekends to get Nathan, and keeping some semblance of order in her father's apartment, wishes for the simplicity of spending a whole day in the hospital and retiring to a hotel bar and a hotel bed. She and Kathy agreed: this is a bad situation and there is no way to do it well, or right, or even to make the best of it. You just do what you have to do and see it through. But this realistic attitude denies recognition of her heroic effort. If only she had one thing less to struggle with. If Clare were toilet trained, if it just would't snow so much, if the grandparents lived in New York to take the kids, if there were day care in the hospital for Clare, for her. If I had only done something or other differently, five or however many years ago this started, I may never have wound up here. If, if, if, there is no end of ifs. We will strangle ourselves with ifs.

And tomorrow everything changes again. Tomorrow we walk out the door into the cold and into the next phase of recovery, of new life. Yesterday I was scared. Today I just want to get on with it. Tomorrow, Jean gets a whole new list of chores, but one thing off the list will be to visit Bob in the hospital. That item gets ticked off tomorrow.

DAY TWENTY-THREE

Sunday. Sandy isn't in. I have Linda today for our first and last shift together. Everything is packed into a small suitcase. I am wearing regular people street clothes, a comfy pair of cargo slacks and a sweatshirt. Underpants feel funny. Jean brought in the Sunday Times, then fell asleep on my bed. Jared decided they had better top off my tank with red cells and platelets so my fantasy of going home for lunch has evaporated. I can't read. I'm watching the Knicks play the Bulls. No one in Boston has the slightest interest in the Knicks. Howie, who is in and out to check my vitals almost every other time the ball changes hands, gave me the strangest look, as if he finally accepted that I really am sick. Every four or five minutes I look at the bag of red blood slowly dripping into me. It takes about an hour and a half per unit, and they are giving me two units. That means I get to look at the bag no less than thirty-six times, not counting glances. I may be anxious about what will happen once I get out, but like the day we came in, now let's just get on with it. Don't make me sit through this whole game.

Finally I'm full of blood and loaded with prescriptions for nausea meds, vitamins, folic acid; with needles, syringes, heparin, and dressing-change kits for care of the Hickman; with instructions all over again from the dietician and the discharge nurse; with the Sunday Times. In the suitcase are packed the photos and cards from friends and family, Sandy's blood count chart, a sheaf of one-page-per-day calendar sheets with notes scribbled on the back, the throwaway camera a friend sent in a couple of days ago, and—for some reason that looks less than optimistic—the lead radiation shields. We're ready. The day has worn on so late, I have a new nurse already. I wish Sandy were here. I could use a good hug from her and a shove into the elevator. We aren't going far; I'll be back to the hospital this week and come up and get my hug then. Visit the floor like any ordinary masked person.

I let Jean touch the elevator button. Hospital bugs on that thing. I wait in the lobby while she goes for the car. Standing at the front entrance, masked and emaciated, I attract the attention of a security guard. He wants to know if he can get me a wheelchair.

"I'm going home," I blurt stupidly through the thick mask.

"Good luck to you, then," he says, checking himself from patting me on the back. I look as if a sneeze will knock me over.

Jean pulls the car to the front door and comes inside. She picks up my suitcase, "It's not heavy, I can . . . "

"No you don't."

And we walk to the door. Just as Sandy said they would, the automatic doors snap open for us, I take a deep breath and walk—no, stride—out of Dana-Farber Cancer Institute and into our car. Car door slammed closed, I whip off the mask.

"Home?" she asks, a little choked.

"I thought we might stop at the Prospect for a quick one on the way. Home."

Getting settled at Jack's. I do everything here in slow motion. Slowly up the stairs from our basement bedroom, slowly to sit, slowly to rise, eat slowly, talk slowly. Speed will only get me in trouble. I'm not going anywhere. I have time. Take it slow and easy.

I'm dead tired. More than yesterday. The apartment is such a challenge. I have all this stuff to watch for and remember. Lini said that the Hickman might be pulled before I go home in a week, but for now I still have it to care for. There's all the diet and toilet stuff to remember. It's as much bringing the hospital home as it is getting out of it. Tomorrow I go back for a CBC and a push of G-csf. Jean won't have to visit me in the hospital, but she'll have to ferry me back and forth. Transfusions will take hours.

But. But. Tonight I sat at an ordinary table, in an ordinary chair, and ate a meal with my family. I don't have to wash dishes, I don't have to clear the table, I don't have to cook for everyone. They want me to stay out of the kitchen all together. We'll see how long that lasts.

I sit on a couch. We talk. I look at last week's newspaper. Today's news is that my lap is on this couch. The phone rings. Jean brings me the receiver. I talk to Judy on the phone, sitting on the couch, turning the pages of the newspaper, thinking about what I will eat next, like any ordinary person back from the grave. I love it. I love being back among my family, even though every time Clare squawks, the phone rings, Jean asks the simplest question, Jack smiles, I start, take a deep breath, and only limply respond. I am so tired I cannot speak another word. But I love it.

WEEK FIVE

The surprise of being out is that I don't feel enough difference. I'm constantly tired, I have so many routines to follow, and I'm a burden on everyone.

The constant cleaning of the toilet and the shower is a royal pain for Jean. Fortunately, Jack has three bathrooms, so the rest of the household can do their business and ignore my hygiene schedule.

The stay-out-of-the-kitchen rule lasted until the second morning. While Jean took Clare to day care, and Jack was off to his office, I made myself a bowl of Wheatena and ate it all by myself. From then on, with no complaint from Jean, I took care of my own breakfasts and now even lunches. It's the least I can do.

I do yoga in the mornings on the same mat now in our cellar bedroom. There is less space here than in the hospital, but I manage. One day, holding my feet together, I saw the big wart on the right foot had turned white. With nothing better to do I scraped most of it off. Bone marrow transplant must be the most expensive way yet to get rid of a wart.

Once I gagged on a pill and threw up all over my bathroom. I haven't thrown up in a couple of weeks and thought I was done with it. I mentioned it to Jared when I went to the clinic. "Your insides have been through a lot," he said. "It will take more than a couple of weeks for them to get back to normal. But don't worry. This will happen."

I went to the clinic every day this week. Sometimes just for a CBC and the G-csf. But a couple of times I spent all day there getting transfusions. I've seen Lini a couple of times and she keeps saying they should be able to pull the Hickman before I go home, but in the meantime, I need blood through it.

The clinic doesn't do regular business on Saturdays, but is open for especially needy cases, most of us just out of transplant. Kathy, whom Jean had introduced me to the day before we left, sat next to her husband Kevin who was slumped in a wheelchair and would not lift his face to say hello. He didn't know me and had no strength to acknowledge my existence. He could see as far as Kathy and that was it. Kathy did recognize me and we chatted a little. Having Kevin out was a whole new burden and she was even more tired than when he was in crisis in the hospital. But she spoke proudly about how she and the staff had pulled him through.

While we waited, another woman wheeled her husband in. The two women recognized each other and began to talk. The second guy looked even worse off than Kevin, who at least responded to Kathy. This guy was just a large lump in a wheelchair. The women talked about how they had to do everything for their men. The second lady was a nurse and had never treated such a patient in her life. Then suddenly I recognized the guy. He was admitted the same day I was and was in the waiting room with the intake nurse just ahead of me. That day he was a large, strapping fellow with a booming voice and enormous enthusiasm for this project. Now all I could recognize was his eyes and nose, otherwise he was transformed into a ghost of his former self. His skin had turned a sickly mahogany color, he must have lost fifty pounds, his voice, his very breath, turned to a pale whisper. Yee gods, did I look like this? I was thrown back in my chair. His wife was already used to it. I couldn't look this awful. Jean had dropped me at the front door. I walked through the lobby under my own steam. I talked to people. I was thin, colorless, and more tired than I had been in the hospital, but compared with these guys, I was doing just fine.

If transplant can so transform you, and there is only a fifty-fifty chance it might cure you, is it worth it? The video Bonnie gave us didn't show any patients one week out. If it could make you so totally apathetic, how could these guys ever get better? How come they were so debilitated and I was at least standing upright? Where did their strength go that some modicum of mine stayed with me? Maybe they were not autologous transplants. Maybe they were older. Who could tell how old they were now. Maybe they had had years of chemotherapy, remission, and relapse. Maybe right this minute I was proving Offit's preference for transplant up front. Maybe I got through it the way I did because for me the medicine wasn't strong enough. In a year they will be cured and healthy and I will still be dealing with disease. But Saturday morning they looked horrible. I don't know what I would have done if Bonnie had showed me these pictures rather than the smiling faces framed in newly opened doors.

Another couple joined us. June was now a few weeks out and much stronger. The five of us who could got to talking about this and that, mostly how hard this process is. We got around to alternative therapies we had either tried or read about. Someone mentioned the guy in New York who claims to cure cancer with cappuccino enemas. Six or seven a day. Kathy and I looked at each other for a moment and I said, "Frankly, I don't know if this is so very much worse." We all laughed and I knew, in spite of feeling dead tired and wanting nothing better than to crawl home to bed, that I was on my way back.

Late one afternoon, while Clare played in the middle of the living room and Jack and Jean sipped their well-earned cocktails, I stared for a long time at a splash of sunlight on a bookshelf. I have never sat on his couch for more than a few minutes on a winter afternoon. It takes more than just a few minutes to track the slow fall of sunlight across the room and down the bookshelf opposite the west window. Now I had the time. Just a thin splash of sunlight, but I kept my eye on it and measured the rotating earth by the fall of the shaft. Then it dimmed as less and less sun shone over the building next door. The little light soon disappeared, and I watched every moment until it did. Then turned back to my pad.

What a marvelous thing that the earth turns and light changes and we don't burn up or freeze to death. It's a wonderful clock, the earth ticking away, whether I'm here to see it or not. Today I can see it, and seeing this little light is enough for one day. The room darkens as the light fades. The long night of supper and chores and bed begins. Come summer's longer days and the sun's higher slant there will be no light on this shelf, and I'll be well and romping and too busy to watch one little light dim.

WEEK SIX

At the end of the first week out, the counts were still not high enough either to go off G or to trust that I won't need transfusions. So the second week continued much the same. Since the clinic is completely closed on Sunday, Lini ordered that I inject myself with G and see what happened. As an outpatient, I had given myself the shots during chemo cycles and had no problem with them. When I came back Monday, the count was up. Lini said when G is injected subcutaneously, the body takes longer to absorb it and the effect lasts longer. She decided to let me keep on shooting myself in the thigh.

The high point of the second week out was my first walk alone outdoors. A small step for mankind, an enormous one for me. I had been walking from the apartment to the car, the car to the hospital, the hospital to the car, and the car to the apartment. But late one afternoon this week while Jean was cooking supper, I decided I wanted to get out, stretch, watch the four o'clock sunset, and get over another hump—just into the village and back. I bundled up for the worst: long johns, sweater and vest under my winter parka, mittens, extra socks, boots, a cowl up over my face; I was ready for the Antarctic with Roald Amundsen.

As soon as I hit the pavement, I turned away from the village. Suddenly I wanted instead to walk the quiet old twisting side streets lined with a mixture of large and small old houses and a few small prewar apartment buildings. The street was plowed, but not down to the pavement, and snow was heaped onto the sidewalks in impassable mounds. I walked down the middle of the street, stepping aside into the snowbank to let the occasional car pass.

As I wandered, I was amazed at just being outside. It's still here. I'm still here. Very simple things caught and held my attention: unpainted clapboard, a colored flag left over from summer, a new baby blue paint job with delicate white detailing on a 19th-century manse. A tiny square, in season a few wrought-iron-fenced trees and benches, now one giant mound of snow.

But to be outside on my own. Free of stale air, of constant concern for my temperature and blood pressure, of the how-are-you looks that, while they show great concern, become tiresome after a while. Free for the moment to roam, to wander and wonder. The simple stuff of life is still here and still works. To take the first walk on a mountain top or a seashore would have been too spectacular. A simple city block was just fine. In the moment, magnificent. I stopped by the little square for a few deep breaths.

A car passed and I smelled it, not the exhaust but the gasoline. If I've ever smelled gasoline from a moving car before, I've forgotten. Or maybe I smell it all the time but have gotten so used to it, it doesn't register; this week everything registers. My first impulse was to turn away and pull my cowl up over my nose against the toxic fumes, but instead, I looked for the exhaust pipe. After the car passed, I marveled at the return of smell and that such a small, even noxious, thing should be a wonder.

The sun was gone, and I had been out longer than either of us expected. When I got back to the house, Jean was anxious. She didn't know where to find me what had happened. I had been away all of forty minutes. I know I would have been worried if I were her—like the first time the kid goes off alone to school. Has to be done. But I had a wonderful time walking around the block in the winter under the setting sun and will do it again. Yes, folks, I'm coming back. But I am tired and will go right to bed after supper.

My little saunter was exhausting.

Nathan was here over the weekend, and we were all hoping that Lini would let me go home, so we could drive back together and he wouldn't have to take the bus alone again. But that was not to be. The white count is rising steadily with the G, but she wants it to get over three thousand before she stops it. The platelets don't seem to be holding, which she says is typical, and the red cells don't hold either, but slowly, steadily drop after each transfusion. She would like to see them stabilize so she can pull the Hickman. That doesn't seem to be happening.

Another cousin called and asked if she could bring over some take-out food. She never cooks and she and her husband must live on the stuff. They dropped a load off once before, while I was in the hospital, because a container of crusty mashed potatoes is still in the fridge. Don't touch leftovers, said the dietician. Not even to throw them away? I told the cousin I couldn't eat any restaurant or take-out food. "But how about the others? They can eat it, can't they?" She was going to do what she was going to do whether it did me any good or not.

They showed up at the apartment with a couple of bags of warmed-over food, one look at which convinced me that it was just as well take-out was against the rules. But it was edible, and Jean was happy not to cook another meal, although for me she had to make something. What do I have to complain about?

As soon as the cousin laid eyes on me, she turned for the door. "We don't want to tire or bother you." But I wanted company and asked them to come in.

"Only just for a minute." But she wouldn't sit down until finally her husband told her to. I have loved my cousin dearly, but she is very stubborn and lays off on others what she feels. "We don't want to disturb you," means—The sight of you disturbs me very much. "We don't want to tire you," means—I'm tired of standing here." Outside of holidays and funerals, we haven't been close in years. She didn't have to come. I was grateful for the company and grateful for the help. I did my best to make her feel welcome and relaxed, and I failed. Or my looks made the task futile.

I can only guess that she smelled death, and it revolted her so. Once I told Judy that I could taste death. But I know now I was exaggerating. I have risked death, yes, but I was not close enough to taste it. I suppose to this cousin I look like death warmed over, but I am not the kiss of death. I may be feathery, but a gentle hug won't crush me. What harm will it do her? I want to squeeze her. Look at me, folks: fighting cancer is not threatening, it is scary as hell. Not fighting is the threat.

WEEK SEVEN

Finally, Lini couldn't keep me any longer. The white count was three thousand, but after transfusions, the platelets and red cells kept sliding. I will have to keep the Hickman, at least for a while.

"If you lived in northern Maine, I wouldn't let you go. But I don't suppose that we can do any better for you than Memorial." But first they topped off my tanks with blood and gave me one last shot of G. Then back up to the floor to get dressing-change kits for the Hickman. Sandy took me to the supply room and filled a shopping bag with everything I would need. She recorded it all into the computer. "For billing, you know. They have been getting very sticky about supplies." I'm just itching to see the bills for this thing. We had another big hug and she was about to send me on my way, when Linda, my nurse the last day, had a question.

"You're from New York, right?"

"Well it seems like a lifetime ago, but yeah."

"And you have a kid in fifth grade in Manhattan, right?"

"Who is pissed off we didn't come home last weekend."

"Well, come here. I have someone for you to meet." Linda walked me to the door of my old room, 1234. "The patient in your bed is Joanne. She says her daughter goes to school with your son."

"You are kidding."

"I don't think so." Joanne came to the window, and we shouted how are yous through the glass and established that indeed our kids were in the same class. I remember Nathan saying that a kid had told the class that her mother was going to the hospital in Boston. But we had no idea she was going to the same hospital, and that Lini was her doctor and she'd wind up in the very same bed. She told me that Nathan had been very helpful in telling her daughter what having a parent in transplant was like—something he has since denied; not the telling part, the very helpful part.

She had just checked in and was about to start TBI. She smiled and waved. I pulled off my skull cap, gave her a salute, shouted, "I warmed up the bed for you," and blew her a kiss.

Back to Sandy for one last hug. "The next time I see you, you'll have hair and be a normal person again."

"Next time I see you, you'll be a mother, which for a while won't feel so normal. Good luck to you too."

As I stood at the desk in the clinic, waiting to check out and have one last goodbye from Lini, I watched Rob Soiffer chat with a hearty young man. The fellow was smiling and full of energy. He had a full head of hair and a full beard. I could tell he was a transplant patient ten or twelve months out. This could be me in a year. If I make it. If I look like I do now in six months, I'm going to be anything but hearty.

Lini wished me luck and shook my hand, but I pulled her toward me. She wasn't getting away without a hug. Then Jean and I walked out of Dana-Farber, stronger but more sober than two weeks ago.

We went to Jack's and packed. I filled an envelope with the calendar pages, the cards and letters that people sent, Sandy's chart of the roller coaster my blood counts have been on, the throwaway camera we hadn't developed yet. I didn't want to carry the lead shields, but didn't want to toss them, so I slid the two glove-wrapped packages into a dresser drawer. We'll be back.

Jean's brother helped us pack the car, more hugs all around and we were off. Nathan was waiting in New York. He asked on the phone what I was going to do about the bathroom on the way. I hadn't thought about it, but he was paying attention. My mouth was still dry from the radiation, no way I'd make the four-hour trip without a pit stop. Just have to be careful.

North of Hartford, I could barely hold it anymore. We pulled into a service area; I put on the mask and backed into the public toilet without touching any handles. I washed carefully, but how was I going to pull open the doors I had pushed? I could simply wait until someone else went ahead and slipstream behind him. But that was going to look a bit strange: this masked character hanging around the men's john, then following some guy out. So I washed my hands again and used the paper towels to open the doors, then quickly threw out the towels when I got to the parking lot. This is the way it is going to be. The world is unsanitary, and I will have to weave my way through it without coming down with some bug that can kill me.

Back in New York, people in our lobby kind of kept their distance, but the doorman rushed to take the bags from Jean. In the mirror facing the street door was a gray, sickly looking older man coming slowly toward me as I walked across the lobby. Oh, shit, no. I hadn't been afraid before to look in the mirror. I even took a picture in the hospital room mirror. But right here, in this mirror, a part of the furniture I passed everyday barely noticing, I wasn't expecting the sight of my cadaverous self. Well, my bald and wizened friend, you have a ways to travel yet.

Our little apartment looked cozy for the moment. A friend had sent her cleaning lady, and the expected grime and mess from six weeks' neglect and a kid's part-time habitation were mercifully erased before we got home. Ah, to lie in my own bed again. But there it is, I wanted first to be back in bed. I was totally exhausted.

Lini ordered that I have blood drawn every third day. Dr. Offit said I should come see him in a week and if I need transfusions to come to Memorial. But in my condition, I don't want to schlep over to the East Side just for a CBC. So I asked Dr. Collens, whose office is a few blocks downtown, to draw the blood. "No problem. However I can be of help."

So two days after I got back, I walked—under my own steam—down the hill to Ninety-sixth Street. There is less snow here and the leftover piles are filthy. But it's familiar old New York, hometown filth, and I'm happy to be back in it. Except for my mask, I am an ordinary pedestrian risking his fool life on the street. Not quite ordinary. Now I wait for the walk sign to change; on the sidewalk, not halfway out into the intersection. For someone just out of the hospital, the short hill up from Ninety-sixth isn't so easy, and by the time I got to his office I was short of breath. The day Dr. Collens put me into the hospital for non-resolving pneumonia, I was short of breath on this hill.

Today he gave me a big hug as soon as he saw me. "You made it. Oh, it's good to see you. Look at you. I'll bet you gave people a fright on the street with that mask."

"This is New York. No one even looked up."

He drew the blood with the surest hands and sent it off to the lab. I would call later to get the results. Instead of going right home I took a get reacquainted detour up Broadway. Ah, these streets. That such grime is so lively. Happy to look the size of an insect from twelve stories up, instead of looking down from a hospital room.

If the counts are low, I'm supposed to call Eugenie to arrange a transfusion. Memorial's rules differ from Dana-Farber's. They transfuse platelets when the count drops below ten thousand, not twenty, and red cells when the hemoglobin is below seven. Of course an outside count won't be sufficient; at Memorial they will have to run their own CBC and type and cross for the blood match. But I'm a post-bone-marrow-cancer patient, the cancer hospital is where I belong. Saving cab rides is false economy.

I think I'm a little stronger this week, but it's hard to tell. I'm as tired and weak as I have ever been in my own apartment. With Nathan in school and Clare in day care or with Jean, I'm alone here much of the time. I draw energy from the empty apartment. Who knows, I might even write a little.

MONTH THREE

Last week I was almost admitted to the hospital with another lung infection. I came down with a cough and then a fever, and Dr. Offit sent me to Dr. Stover. She and Gail ordered a chest X-ray, blood tests, and a sputum sample. They were able to diagnose klebsiella and put me on oral antibiotics. "But if this doesn't work," Dr. Stover said, "you'll have to be admitted. We can't do much without a white count." During the exam, Gail asked lots of questions about the transplant. She had not been entirely convinced that transplant was the right move for me, and now she seemed relieved that I had made it as well as I had. She reminded me that I have other caregivers now to rely on. When she put her cold hand on my shoulder, I jumped. "You still have cold hands."

"Sorry."

"Still is good. Your hands are cold, still; I'm here, still."

Now I'm back in the day hospital where Elizabeth, my chemo nurse, is giving me a transfusion and treating me with fond care. She gives me Benadryl in case of an allergic reaction to the blood or maybe just to put me to sleep. I just woke up. Elizabeth is very proprietary and not pleased when I have to come in on her day off. I'm touched. But I wish my marrow would start making its own blood, thank you very much, and I wouldn't have to come in at all. But Elizabeth is going to see me through. "We're beating this sucker" is her line, and I remind her of it when I get the chance.

We've settled into a routine. I see Eugenie twice a week for blood counts. If I'm OK, I go home. If I need a transfusion, she draws the type and cross so that Elizabeth will have the blood first thing the next morning. Saves waiting time. Eugenie works for several lymphoma doctors and I've now sat in just about every waiting room in the outpatient clinic while she gets the results. This waiting for the counts to come back is driving me a wee bit crazy. Lini thought the Hickman would be pulled weeks ago, and there is still no sign that the marrow can sustain a red count. If I weren't so tired all the time, I would be furious.

Yesterday, tired or not, I came very close to losing it altogether. While I was waiting for Eugenie, two men in leather sport coats sat opposite me. One was old enough to be the other's father, or uncle maybe. I couldn't tell which was the patient; maybe they were both waiting for someone else. Other people's stories interest me. Sometimes we swap tales; other times I just listen and watch. There's a truck load of drama in these rooms.

As I watched, this older leather guy, with a sweeping gesture that took in the whole lot of us waiting patients, announced in a loud foreign accent, "Look. You see all these people. They are all dying." Just like that, with the flick of his wrist, he killed us off. I flared. I sputtered. I almost got up and punched him.

I am not dying. I am surviving. I am going to make it. Who the hell are you to pronounce me dead in the waiting room?

If I had hit him, I would have had righteousness on my side. I mean, look at me. "A near cadaver in the cancer hospital rises slowly from his barely warm seat and weakly, but dramatically, socks macho man, who survives the punch but not the wound it causes."

I mean, who the fuck is he, doctor doom? His accent was Eastern European. Maybe downwind of Chernoble there is little hope, and I am not gloating over the fact that I don't live there, but what does it do for this man to condemn the rest of us? Does it build him up? By this gesture does he convince himself that his illness is not deadly? Or is he waiting for his nephew to die? Does he think his gloom will somehow encourage the poor kid next to him? He's immortal, right? And we poor suffering cancer-ridden slobs are doomed? And the jerk is going to be oh so inconvenienced when he has to ride the elevator down to York Avenue and stand on the street corner with the crowd of hospital workers and patients with their half dozen IV bags dangling from poles in order to smoke his next cigarette. Entering this no-smoking hospital you have to cross a picket line of smokers. I can understand the patients—their butt is their last friend—but the staff? To work in a cancer hospital and stand in front of it smoking? What is the meaning of this? But this creep sitting across from me, he's immortal; he's some minor god who exterminates a handful of sick people simply to convince himself he is alive. I'm going off the deep end. Where the hell is Eugenie?

OK, maybe the guy is Bosnian. The suffering he has seen makes us appear coddled. In his country there isn't enough medicine to care for the people who are savable, children who could survive to live long lives. He says to himself—Look at this cushy waiting room and these smart assistants, these expensive doctors and their tests up the ying yang, all for a bunch of stiffs. Look at that skinny Jewish guy sitting opposite us, the one all alone with that mask on and no hair, his yellow skin. In Bosnia (or Somalia or South Africa or Tibet) we would leave such a creature out in the woods to die. It is obscene to spend all this money. We have nothing for the children, how can they possibly afford to give anything to this guy. All these people are dying, and they should hurry up and die already and stop trying to make up for the waste of life everywhere else in the world. Then maybe this place won't be as depressing with them out of it, and they won't take up so much of my doctor's time.

I hate the guy and still want to punch him for making me feel guilty on top of everything else. He thought he was being realistic. He can flush his realism where he does the rest of his business. He can keep his dirty remarks to himself. He can drop dead himself already. C'mon, Eugenie, get me out of this. Don't make me stew any longer. I'm sitting somewhere else.

I've seen people make scenes in these waiting rooms. Some guy last week was screaming that the urgent care had misdiagnosed his wife, and she had to go to a local ER, and now she was back, and he was going right to the president and would sue. He wanted to see the doctor. He wanted to see the head of this and the chief of that. He was going right to the president. The social worker couldn't deal with the guy and called Eugenie. Out she came—tall, smart, black, proud, take-no-nonsense—and she handled the guy. One and only one apology she gave him. He wanted immediate action. She explained that before they could do anything for his wife, who was sinking deeper and deeper into the sofa, they needed the blood tests back. Eugenie was holding a bag with the blood tubes.

"Look, sir. If you don't let me bring these to the lab, it's only going to take longer. And as soon as we know what we are looking at, we will act. We will not run off half-cocked and treat your wife for something she may not have. Would that be smart?"

"But she is sick. She needs attention now."

"Sir, she's getting it. I have a whole room full of sick people," Eugenie caught my eye, "who need attention. Sue if you want to, that's your business. We are doing what we can."

The guy had a righteous point. I know mistakes get made, and to lose control of your care is as anxiety provoking as the disease itself, but I was proud of Eugenie at that moment. This lady takes no bull and she's my nurse.

Mr. Leather Jacket shut up and looked at a magazine. Eugenie finally reported my counts, and the word was to come back tomorrow for transfusion. I left the hospital still pumped and not ready for the ride home. I walked toward the park and when I came to Hunter, decided to stop in at the dance department and say hello. I'd designed the lighting for their concerts for eleven years, until this spring. With the mask back on, I found Jana, the chair, and she gave me a big hug. We talked about me first and then about her semester and the concert that was in rehearsal now. Wouldn't I like to go down to the theater and say hello? I thought they might not be so tickled to see me, but they were. I may look a sight, but I have survived, and here I am walking the streets of New York. People like to see that. The disease is a real pisser, but just by walking in off the street I show that there is a hope of beating it.

I wasn't prepared for their enthusiasm. Family and friends were living with this as I was, day by day. You look a little better. You don't look quite so good. Here they were both shocked and pleased.

"Is there anything we can do?"

"Give platelets at Memorial," I said. "It's right down the street."

"Tell us how."

Then I walked slowly and gingerly out onstage. Last spring, the long renovation of the theater was finished, and I had lit the very first performance when it reopened. I would come to rehearsals directly from chemo. Once one of the students noticed the bandage on my hand and said: "You had a blood test. Are you all right?"

"Yeah. I'm OK." I was OK at the moment. Should I have given her my story while she was warming up to dance?

I went out into the house and sat at the design table. We were only twenty minutes behind schedule, and my attention wasn't needed just then. I sat back and watched the young people, some rehearsing, others chatting or studying, all the quiet hubbub before a rehearsal gets underway. They seemed so young, so free—Bob, you are the only one, I said to myself. The only one here with cancer. But in an instant I was brought up short—You don't know that. Whether they know they have it or not, you probably aren't the only one. Hidden in one or more of these bodies is the disease. And surely out of the forty or fifty people in the theater you will not be the only one for long.

But today everyone looked fairly healthy and glad to see me, which helped to no end after Mr. Leather Jacket's tantrum. Or was the tantrum mine?

MONTH FOUR

I'm back in the hospital, lymphoma service, two beds, no roommate. And it's my birthday I'm spending inside. Don't ask how old, I told you already back at Farber.

I came down with a fever. The rule is, you must call with a fever of 101 or higher. But Eugenie said if it's 100.5 and has been rising, call. Even with the rule, when to call is a nerve-racking decision. It goes like this. I don't feel too well, I feel warm, I take my temp, it's 99. Should I call? I don't want to call. The rule is 101. I don't want to start with the blood draws, tests, X-rays, exams, the whole list. I don't want to go over to the East Side, the hospital side of town. I want whatever it is to go away. Then the fever does go down. See, I did the right thing. Nothing to it. The fever goes up. I should have called, but it still isn't high enough. The fever goes up and down for a couple of days until finally it hits 101, and I call, and Eugenie says come in, and I heave a sigh and flag a cab.

Late afternoon yesterday, Friday, I found her in a clinic I had never been to before, where she was covering for the nurse of a different lymphoma doctor. She took my vitals and drew a CBC and blood cultures. No need to fingerstick because nurses are permitted to draw from the Hickman. Anyone can draw out, but only nurses and doctors are allowed to inject anything back into a patient, and without injecting heparin, the line becomes clogged and useless. She sent the vials to the lab and we waited together to see if I needed a transfusion and for Dr. Offit to call back about the fever.

Eugenie had had a rough day and was only now getting to eat lunch. I was the only patient so I sat with her while she ate. It was kind of pleasant and homey just to chat with her while she downed her now cold something parmigiana out of a styrofoam box.

But a call came in and she was back at work with her mouth full. A patient had been sent home with a prescription for G-csf but no needles because his daughter thought the visiting nurse was going to give him the shots, but the visiting nurse hadn't shown up. Eugenie asked to speak to the patient, but he spoke only Chinese. She didn't know the patient because he belonged to the nurse she was covering for. Could the daughter give him the shot? Could he give himself the shot? (I'm an old hand at shooting myself with G. What's the big deal here? But I remembered my own words: everybody has to find his own way through this mess. For this guy, giving himself a shot was not on the route.) Eugenie spent a good half hour arranging for this person to come into the urgent care that night to have a nurse give him his G, but then the daughter refused to come to Manhattan this late in the day. Without a chart, without knowing the family or the patient, without a word of Chinese, Eugenie finessed the situation: the daughter would bring the patient into the urgent care first thing in the morning. In the meantime, Eugenie left a hefty voice-mail trail for the attending. I remembered the guy in the leather jacket. Not even this patient, seemingly incapable of a simple act for his own care, is condemned, not by Eugenie.

The CBC results came back, and, yes, I did need a red cell transfusion, but the day hospital was about to close so I would have to be transfused in the urgent care. The fever was not high enough to admit me, and there were no other symptoms. She left word with Dr. Offit and sent me downstairs. Urgent care would take hours to give me the blood. I wouldn't be out of the hospital until nine, if they let me out. And I wanted to go home. Now off the post-transplant food regimen, birthday cake, even birthday salad, was on my menu.

While I waited at urgent care, Dr. Offit called and suggested I go on G-csf for a week to boost the white count while fighting whatever it was I was fighting. "Go home when you're finished taking your blood and call me on Monday." Go home sounded good. And a little after nine I climbed into a cab. The urgent care unit is not a pleasant place. People wind up here for a variety of reasons ranging from not so good to terrible. To walk out on my own steam was fine with me.

But the next morning, just as we were getting our breakfast, a doctor I had never heard of before called from a lab. I had an infection and had to come back to the urgent care right away.

"How do you know? What are you talking about?"

"I'm a pathologist. Something is growing in one of the cultures taken yesterday."

"What is growing?"

"It doesn't matter exactly what it is, it isn't supposed to be there. You have to go in and start antibiotics right away."

"Can I have my breakfast? It's my birthday."

"Then go right after breakfast."

"OK."

"Happy birthday."

"You said it."

I sat down with the family to what was supposed to be a celebration—I have lived another year, and what a year it has been. I felt terrible about going back to the hospital and scared shitless that something potentially awful was the matter with me. Who was this doctor? It must be serious when they call you directly from the lab.

Jean served up breakfast. She spooned some of my scrambled egg onto the table and then scooped it up onto my plate.

"You want me to eat that now?" I snapped. She slammed the spatula on the table, switched plates, and served me again from the frying pan. Who could eat now? Happy birthday, Daddy.

At urgent care, the doctor was very annoyed to find out that I had been in last night and they hadn't admitted me.

"The fever is only one hundred. You can't give me antibiotics?"

"Oh, we'll give you antibiotics all right, but IV. For an infection in your line you have to come into the hospital, there's no question. But what they sent you home for . . . it's ridiculous."

"What is this infection called?" Gail had told me about the last one and that I likely picked it up in the hospital.

"Do you have a degree in microbiology?" the guy asked.

"No."

"Then whatever I tell you will have no meaning. Wait here while I do the paperwork to get you a bed."

Who the hell am I to want some information? To this character, I was the carrier, the petri dish, for this bug. I wasn't used to this attitude from doctors. Either I have been very lucky or this guy has especially bad bedside manners, or both.

They didn't have a bed right away, so they started the antibiotic in the urgent care room. Vancomycin. Later I found out that vanco is a top—or end—of-the-line antibiotic. Finally, I was taken to the lymphoma floor, same place I received the first chemo fourteen months ago.

This truly sucks to be back in the hospital. I thought I was feeling a little better.

I have been very careful taking care of the Hickman, injecting it with heparin and rebandaging the site every other day. Memorial has a different protocol: change more often but not with a sterile kit. Maybe that's how it got infected.

The question now is: should they try to save the line or pull it and start again? If pulling it would solve the problem, go ahead. But because I have a fever, the infection is in the blood stream and I still need the full course of vancomycin whether the Hickman is pulled or not. There is no sign that I will soon be free of transfusions and the catheter makes that process much easier. The nurses love the Hickman. They don't want to stick you any more than you want to get stuck. So I am all for trying to save the Hickman and so is the attending, Dr. Farber. While the line infection is the focus of our talk, he also wants to know about the transplant and my general health. As Offit said once, "All medicine comes down to this." When the doctors have seen how rough it can be, they have a kind of awe—perhaps sometimes grudging—for the survivors. Farber (I should ask him if he is any relation) is a little freer with his respect. He wants to know. This is a teaching hospital, and the teaching works in many directions. I'm going to try and get some sleep now. Back tomorrow.

The infection appears to be responding to the antibiotic. Dr. Farber thinks I will be able to leave and get infusion therapy at home. This is great news. I want out of the hospital and the sooner the better.

The visiting nurse visited me, to show her face and to do the paperwork to get me the home care. And what a gorgeous face it is. The thought of her visiting me for the next however many days it takes is not so entirely unpleasant. The social worker is checking the insurance company to make sure they cover the home care. If not, I will have to stay in the hospital. Home care isn't cheap, but a small fraction of inpatient care. The insurance company would be totally insane not to cover it. Don't get me started on insurance now, but when I get some energy back, I'll give you an earful.

Not every moment this month has been spent coming and going from the hospital. We went to a restaurant. Following the rules, we went during the middle of the afternoon when the little bistro was nearly empty. Table clothes, cloth napkins, silverware, the light off the street softened by lace, a nice late lunch. Jean had a glass of wine; I drank seltzer, the preferred substitute of recovering everybodies. I ate a fresh mozzarella something with basil and sundried tomatoes. Tasty, refined. Hey, folks, I'm back in the world.

My sister came from Israel and came to Memorial with me and donated platelets and was tissue-typed for bone marrow donation. Even though we knew I won't use hers, she still wanted to have this done. It was very good of her.

Three nights in the hospital, and I'm back home to finish the course of vancomycin on my own. The visiting nurse doesn't actually give me the medicine, but has taught me how to do it myself. She'll come every three days to draw blood for cultures that should chart the retreat of the infection. Since I also still have to check my counts every three days, I asked if she couldn't also draw blood for the CBC. To my surprise this turned out to be "No problem." We'll see how the insurance company can mess up the bill on this one.

Here's what my beautiful nurse has taught me. I'm amazed that I paid any attention to her words. (Repeating what she's taught me is good practice, but you can skip this part. It has needles in it.) The first step is to take a single dose of vanco out of the refrigerator a half hour early and hang it on the IV pole. This I could do on the first try. When it warms up a little, attach the tubing—new tubing in the morning, used again at night—and prime it with the solution. Then attach the needle to the end of the tubing and swab the Hickman port with Betadine and alcohols. One port in the morning and the other at night to make sure the antibiotic makes contact inside both ports. With the clean port in one hand and the tube in the other, I pull the cap off the needle with my teeth and insert it into the port. Then start the solution flowing with the wheely job that crimps the hose shut. I'm telling you she'll make a nurse out of me yet. The crucial part is not to touch either the clean port or the needle to anything because that could introduce bugs. Once the stuff is running into me, I can do what I like, as long as I can get there pushing the IV pole. I take a little nap or lay down to read. Once or twice I've wheeled the thing to the table to eat supper. When the infusion is finished, I have to flush the line with saline and heparin. Oh, the whole thing is a pain, but it sure beats the hospital, which beats an infection.

For the kids this is an awakening. It's not Dad in the hospital, but the hospital has come home with Dad. I tell them it's better to be here than there. But maybe they don't think so. The infusion doesn't take more than forty-five minutes. And I'm around the house, I can help take care of them. With a mask on I can go to Clare's day care and bring her home. I wear a mask and gloves to change her diapers, but she's old enough now to be trained. I talk about big girls using the toilet. Somewhere in her mind she knows that toilet training is something she can do to help. What it might mean for her to have been toilet trained by a Daddy in a mask, I don't know, and I can't give it great thought. If this thing is done with love, pride, and tolerance, it really won't much matter that Daddy has tubes sticking out of his chest. Or is this just what my mother did—treat the illness as normal? (Well, it has become a new kind of normal.) Or did she simply do the best she could? What a thing to stick in the story of a bone marrow transplant: toilet training my daughter. But here we are, another thing that has to be done. As soon as she is ready for it, I say go for it. We'll survive the consequences.

The antibiotic has cleaned out the line infection and the guy from the infusion company has picked up the leftover equipment. Sorry to say goodbye to the nurse, but easy come, easy go. So where are the blood counts? Dogging around doing nothing. Offit's new fellow, Dr. Bromberg, did a bone marrow biopsy to see what is going on there. She showed it to me as she put the biopsy into the test tube. It was white. It's supposed to be bloody. And the result came back nothing. Negative for lymphoma, negative for blood. Empty. Yikes. I talked to Richard. He asked if Dana-Farber had given me back all the marrow they had harvested. I never heard anything about saving out some marrow. He implied that the marrow lacked sufficient stem cells. But clearly there were some. I had a white count even without G, and though the platelets dipped close to ten thousand, they kept coming back into the teens and twenties. So what's going on?

Offit doesn't quite know, but we sat down in conference with Dr. Bromberg and Eugenie. Jackie had worked on Memorial's transplant team and they gave half the dose of acyclovir that I was taking under the Farber protocol. Maybe the acyclovir depressed the counts. Why not try stopping or cutting down on that?

"OK, good," said Dr. Offit, "this is what we do. One, we try Dr. Bromberg's experiment. It won't work, but maybe we'll be surprised. Stop acyclovir for two weeks. When this does nothing, we'll put you back on a reduced dose. Don't want you coming down with chicken pox. Then we try erythropoietin to stimulate red cell production. Your kidneys are making plenty of it already, which is both good and bad. Good because it means that your kidneys are

OK, bad because it doesn't explain what's the matter with your blood production. Now this will take at least three months."

"Three months?"

"Yeah, you can't expect it to work right away like G. You give yourself a shot every three days. We step you up and then step you down and see what happens."

"And what next?"

"Well there are worse things than giving yourself a shot twice a week. Look at diabetics." Of course he's right; after what I have been through this will be minor. But in the moment I am not at all pleased to hear that I might have to take this stuff for the rest of my days.

"If erythro doesn't work we try immunoglobulin shots, but that's way down the road and we don't want to go that route if we don't have to. In the meantime, go away and don't take acyclovir."

Anything to stay out of the hospital.

MONTH FIVE

Our luck has begun to change. While I was in the hospital and Jean back on campus, she asked to be considered for college housing. Her new role in her department will mean more time on campus. If we live in New York she will commute more and be away just when we need her at home. Nathan will be going into middle school and Clare is old enough for nursery school, which the college provides faculty and staff. It's a decent time to move. I'm not about to work any time soon and can do with a change. And what if I don't make it? Seeing the family settled near Jean's work will ease my mind and hers too. But in my condition, the prospect of looking for a house, to rent even, seems daunting. The college can help.

The college has just acquired an old house at the far end of campus. It needs a lot of work, but they've already started. To move from three rooms in Manhattan to eight in the country will be a shock, but to breathe country air and retreat from the garbage trucks and constant grind of New York will be a pleasure.

I've been enormously frustrated because the counts are only very slowly improving, and no one can tell me why. The day Nathan graduated from elementary school, I thought I might see the classmate's mother who took over my bed at Dana-Farber. But the auditorium was packed with people, so I called her later that day. We had a nice chat and commiserated about how tired we still get. She was shocked to hear I still have the Hickman. Hers was pulled soon after she got out. "I don't know what I'd do if I were still transfusion dependent."—Yikes, what's the matter with me then? I better do something.

I went back to Sandy, the healer. Again I can't tell you what she did exactly or how it works, but I've seen her a few times and will continue for a while. Something is moving. What harm can meditating and visualizing the bone marrow's making cells do?

The lowest platelet counts are finally more than high enough to free me from platelet transfusions. I'm seeing Bob Abramson again. We talked a few times since I've been home and agreed that until the platelet count was sufficient, I had better stay away from acupuncture. The first time he laid eyes on me, he gave me a big hug. "So you've been to the top of the mountain," he said, beaming.

"And lived to tell the tale," I replied.

The animus many holistic healers feel toward Western medicine is thick and famous. They bad-mouth doctors and cheer when you do some alternative, any alternative, as long as the medicine does not need an Rx and the practitioner is anything but an MD. Bob has none of this. He always notes what the other doctors are saying and views Chinese and Western medicine as complementary approaches. He does not criticize the Western because he now practices Chinese medicine. "When you need the Western approach, thank God for it," he says and tells a story of an old Chinese doctor speaking before a Western audience. A woman asked what he recommended for brain tumors, and the doctor replied, "Surgery." This wasn't the answer she expected and was not satisfied.

"But what did people in ancient China do?" she asked.

"They died," replied the doctor.

For some reason, either Sandy's internal work, or acupuncture, or erythropoietin, or just time, or a mixture of them all, the period between red cell transfusions is getting longer. It looks as if I might have a chance at normalcy.

With Dr. Offit and Eugenie I brought up the issue of pulling the Hickman. "We can't be sure what will happen, but you might be on the road. Eugenie, what do you think?"

"Let me see your arms." I rolled up my sleeves. "You have veins. We could transfuse you without the Hickman if we had to."

"OK, this is what we do," said Offit. "Next time you need a transfusion we'll give it to you through the catheter and then pull it out. Eugenie will set it up with a surgeon. No sense in making you come in an extra time. Fair enough?" I would have preferred them to pull it then and there. I'm sick of taping plastic bags to my chest every time I take a shower or I want to go swimming, which you can't do with a central line in. But I see his point. Get one more transfusion into me and pretty soon my system will take over and make its own blood, thank you very much.

We plan to move in time to settle before the semester starts. One weekend we visited the new house in the midst of its renovations. The carpenters have a lot left to do, but we could see how living here will change our lives, and we are ready for it. Late in the day, I went back upstairs for one last look at the bedrooms. From where I will sleep I could see the sunset. What a change from our Manhattan cave. And what a comfort, after all this time spent in bed, that now I was moving to a bed with a view.

MONTH SIX

But here I am in the hospital again. We were planning to take a load up to the house when I spiked a fever. I suspected another line infection and at the urgent care they drew cultures. This time I started talking immediately about pulling the line. The attending on service, Dr. O'Brien, called, and Offit agreed, get that line out. Yesterday, they rousted up a surgical resident. He shot my chest with lidocaine and cut and pulled and tugged at the thing that for six months had been a part of my body. Because I was bleeding, he had me transfused with platelets through an IV in my arm while he yanked on the one in my chest. I tried to practice deep breathing. Three or four more times he shot me with lidocaine before the tube finally broke free. He was sweating. He explained that it is designed with a collar near the surface of the chest and that my tissue had grown tight around the collar making it hard to pull out. Usually, if the thing were infected it would slide right out, he said, so he will be surprised if my fever were caused by a line infection. But in any case, he had the intern snip off the bloody inside tip of the white tube and send it to the lab. This little hunk of plastic I had been carrying around in my chest for months. Now it belongs to pathologists. Goodbye. Hope we don't see the likes of you again. But thanks just the same.

None of the tests and cultures has shown anything yet. O'Brien doesn't know why I had a fever. Maybe we won't know. Maybe these fevers come and go among post-transplant types. I am free of the Hickman, and I don't even need a red cell transfusion; the last one was three weeks ago. Stay one more night, O'Brien said. Why?

"To be doubly sure there is nothing else the matter." Then he looked at his entourage—a fellow, a resident, and an intern—and said, "And because I'm the smartest guy in the room, and I say stay." Who were we to argue? So here I am.

I have a roommate now. The kid is in terrible shape. He's eighteen and has some rare and very fast moving lymphoma that is gobbling up his platelets. He was treated at home until this new platelet thing started, and his doctor said the only place for him was Memorial. His parents are in and out of the room constantly. The poor kid can barely focus, but he can thrash around and sit and yell. He is very agitated. Last night he was in intensive care and today they gave him a bronchoscopy.

It's nearly midnight. They keep coming and going for Bruce, my roommate. The staff want to move him back to the ICU, but he doesn't want to go. I walk out into the hall and talk to his folks. His mother says he won't move because he had such a horrible time there last night, and he has confused the place with the cause.

His folks are a portrait in coping. They know this may be it, but hold onto any hope they can. Just months ago, the kid was having a fine time skiing when he broke his leg. It wouldn't heal, and they found out the reason was lymphoma. His mother says—call it desperate, but I know what she means—that the broken leg probably saved Bruce's life. If he lives.

He calms down and I go back to bed, but the quiet doesn't last and I go back out to the corridor. My night nurse, rushing to my roommate, takes one look at me and says, "Him, we have to get him another room." I'm glad someone noticed, though I'm feeling pretty well, and I'm kind of the only one here for the parents. The staff are desperately trying to convince the son to go to the ICU. But he's eighteen, no longer a minor, and neither his parents nor anyone else can force treatment on him. Every few minutes one of them goes back in and says a few words to him or just stands and watches. He must think ICU is the end of the line, and if he can stay out of it he'll be OK. He is confused, but not confused enough to be declared incompetent.

His father, to change the subject and to be polite, asks about me. While no story in the cancer hospital is routine, no one who is standing and breathing and going home tomorrow—and maybe not coming back—has a story even remotely as painful as this man's is right now. But when I tell him that while my recovery has been harder and longer than anyone predicted, I show no signs of cancer, he brightens. "Once they get Bruce through this they want him to have a transplant. We didn't know what to think. But look at you. This is good news." If.

Finally, Bruce asks if he can go to the ICU in the bed he is lying in and not shift to a gurney. No one is about to cross him on this one. Absolutely. Stay in bed and we'll wheel you down. I watch as they take him to the elevator. He is having a great deal of difficulty breathing. I give his folks quick hugs and return to my now quiet room. I stare at the space where his bed was. A water pitcher on the night table, some syringe wrappers on the floor, an overflowing waste basket. That's it.

You do what you can. Bruce's father is a volunteer fire fighter in his home town. When the word went out that his son was in dire straights and needed platelet transfusions almost hourly, the fire squad organized a phone tree to get neighbors to donate platelets. In one day they carpooled twenty-five people into New York to donate.

I'm cabbing home again, feeling OK and ready to get on with life after a catheter. On my way out, I stopped at the ICU waiting room and found Bruce's mother. Bruce was having so much trouble breathing they told him he would be more comfortable on a ventilator. Maybe so. She did seem a bit relaxed to have him in intensive care. She urged me to go in and visit him.

"Really, it's OK to visit," as if her son were the reason I came into the hospital. But I drew the line. I didn't think the hospital ICU was the place for me to visit.

Should I have asked for their address and phone number? I didn't. I had my own disease to watch out for. I did what I could.

MONTH SEVEN

My tale of woe, measured in bulk of pages, will never amount to much of a stack compared to the pile of bills. The battle has been joined for months and there is no end in sight. If at all possible, the health insurance company will screw up. I have come to believe that these are not mistakes; rejection is what they are in business to do. Strictly speaking, health insurance is a misnomer; we have none in this country. What we have is sickness insurance. Health, no. The auto insurance company does not insure you against safe driving, but against accidents. The so-called health insurance company is not in the business of delivering health care or of making health care affordable or even of making sickness care affordable. They are in the business of making money. They charge you premiums, and when you want some health care back, they are loathe to part with your money. We live under the illusion that they are taking a risk. It is not so much a risk as a bet. They take our money betting that we will stay healthy, and the only way we can cash in on the bet is to get sick. No sane person would call this health insurance. And the kicker is that when we prove to them that under their contract we are indeed sick, and they have to pay these hospital bills, and they do pay, they turn around and raise the premiums, up the ante. So much for risk taking.

I sound ungrateful. I am not. Our family is not in an HMO and in time the company is paying the bills, most of them. But I am sick. Why when I am weak and vulnerable do I also have to take on the enormous task of keeping the insurance company honest? I work two part-time jobs here: one is staying out of the hospital, and the other staying on the phone to the insurance company. On paper I am making a small fortune at my work, but the family doesn't see a dime in cash.

And the biggest nut, the Dana-Farber inpatient bill, I simply don't worry about. The day before the harvest, a nice woman from Farber called and asked for all our insurance information that I had long ago given another financial officer. Somehow or other my case had "snuck up" on her and she had to get me OK'd by the insurance company in very short order. Trying to help, I gave her the name of the insurance doctor who I was told was supposed to approve the procedure. Him she didn't need, she had her own contacts. "Does this mean I might not be transplanted?"

"Oh, no no no. Don't worry. It just means I have to do some fancy footwork."

She must have danced up a storm because the inpatient bill, nearly six figures of it, has been paid. All but seventy-five dollars for Hickman dressing kits I took home. "Should I have to pay for them?"

"Claims for medical equipment used at home should be submitted as outpatient claims, sir."

"Aye, Aye. I'll have my assistant get right on it." Rule one: never pay a bill just because someone asks you to. Appeal.

But claims for other services have not been so simple. Take the ambulance. Remember the six trips across the street to Brigham and Women's for TBI? That bill didn't go to the insurance company but came to me. I was floored. The total was almost three grand. With no credible explanation, the insurance company decided they should pay only about half. They thought that it was OK to ride an ambulance to the hospital six times in three days, but a patient ought to be able to snag his own ride home. I called the ambulance company for the appropriate codes and the insurance company to make sure they understood why I had to ride so often. The insurance company came up with another big check covering most of the total. The explanation of benefits was so convoluted it took me a day to figure it out, but I had no intention of paying the ambulance company more than my insurance company thought was proper. (See how I shift allegiances when it suits me. Rule two: go with the better deal. Remember Goneril and Regan?)

The insurance company balked at paying a $25.00 per ride mileage charge. Mileage? The distance traveled for all twelve trips could not have been more than one and a half miles, total. I couldn't fault the insurance company on this one and made my case against outrageous overcharging to the ambulance company. They stopped charging me late fees, stopped dunning me, stopped sending me bills altogether. I got no reply, I just never heard from them again. What burns me up is why I, with an insurance company and a hospital finance department, have in the end to take lonely guerilla action against America's rising health costs. It's a nasty job but someone has to do it, and considering where I would be without these services, I'm happy to shoulder the burden.

Not happy, exactly, but I do get a charge out of the struggle. I work hard to get good medical care. I try to be understanding and personal with my caregivers. But with the insurance company it's no holds barred, full battle stations, attack with any means necessary. Shoot first, ask questions later. Whatever it takes. I am not for a minute above hauling out my long sob story in desperate anger. "Look lady (Why are all the customer service reps women?), I just had a bone marrow transplant, OK? That's what this sea of claims is for. Now if you think you can go through this procedure without psychotherapy, be my guest. But if you think I have the energy for this petty "usual and customary" business . . . this is ridiculous. I am a sick man."

"You sound fairly energetic to me, sir."

"Yeah, and along with everything else this insurance company is doing to me, I heartily resent spending my one good hour a day on the phone to you. Not you. It. I'm sure at home you are a lovely person, and I hope you have someone waiting for you there who will listen sympathetically when you complain about this raving bone marrow guy you had to deal with today. But in the meantime, get the company to cover these charges in full."

Of course we reached what they call the stop loss, the point at which you've paid so much that the company starts paying in full. Sort of. They still hit us with "usual and customary," and they still make "mistakes" with the deductible, with my name, Jean's name, her social security number, the address, what they cover, and what they don't cover.

Like the home care. The nurse had to draw blood from the Hickman every third day to track whether the antibiotic was doing its job. The Hickman has two ports, so each time she drew blood there were two identical tests. The insurance company is treating these as duplicate charges for the same test. The lab is trying to help convince them, but in the meantime, they have dunned me.

Who needs this? Sick people? The well are busy working when the ladies of the phone bank come on duty. I sound as if I feel entitled to care. I do, don't you? But I'm doing my job here. I took my medicine, and now I'm following the trail of bills wherever it leads, conscientiously, immediately, and as energetically as I can. So they should stop giving me a hard time.

They also give me, I have to admit, a guilt free opportunity to vent. I grab it with both fists and a shrill whine. But don't tell them. I'm sure they'll figure out some way to bill me for it.

MONTH EIGHT

Slowly and in dribs and drabs, we are moving into our new house. We're not giving up the apartment right away, but between stuff we've had in storage, stuff Jean has had in the apartment she rented near campus this year, and furniture my father no longer needs since his move, we have household goods enough to at least camp here comfortably.

Just in case life might actually be going our way for a while, they, it, the fates, gave us a scare over asbestos. This is the kind of thing that can happen to anybody moving into a renovation, but the way it happened to us seemed so much like getting the cancer diagnosis, it was sickening.

I found a hunk of heating pipe half wrapped in asbestos near the cellar door. If this was how the job was going, where else in the house would we find asbestos? The manager agreed immediately to remove the stuff. Asbestos is bad news, and looking for information about it is like learning about cancer: you do it when you need to and already are scared. Once the pipe wrapping was removed, we were supposed to have an air quality test, a biopsy of the air. They do two kinds: one for any kind of fiber in the air, and a much more expensive test specifically for asbestos. If the air doesn't have much fiber, you don't need the other test.

The results from the first test were borderline. New York has a more rigorous standard than the EPA; in another state the result would have been negative. But getting the news was like hearing the results of the bronchoscopy: you have something the matter, we can't say exactly what, and we need more tests. My knees buckled, my eyes went out of focus, and my stomach dropped to the floor. I've been here before.

Why are they doing this to me? Don't they know what I've been through? Don't they know I've saved up a lifetime of chips? That I have earned a handful of get-out-of-jail cards? This is so clearly unfair, stupid, and wrong. Someone out there has it in for me. And I am not going down again. I asked the air quality guy a armload of questions, the likes of which he was unused to hearing from a customer. He recommended we not return to the house until it was re-cleaned or the other test run. We abandoned the house while a different company reran the first test. A week later, whatever fiber had been in the air—possibly from laying carpet—was gone. More phone calls and we decided to have the expensive test done on the dirtiest sample collected. No asbestos. We heaved a sigh and rented a truck.

Why do I bother you with this? Only to say that bone marrow transplantation does not bestow any special immunity, exemption, or dispensation. You can wind up in jail, or get hit by a bus, just like anybody else. All you get for this enormous effort is more life. Life with all its shocks and heartaches. Considering that I could be dead, I'll take the deal.

I'm lying awake early in the morning. The sun is just up and striking the tops of the pine trees I see out the bedside windows. The morning is cool and the sheets are crisp. Jean is sound asleep next to me. A gentle breeze has come up and the pine bows are swaying lightly. What a lovely way to wake up. What a beautiful place, fresh air, no garbage trucks, only an occasional car on the road, a view across a wide field beyond the pines. An aching freshness.

Yee gods, is this it? OK. It's late summer, not spring. The trees are pines, not maples, but here I am in bed on a pleasant morning, surrounded by trees. What I am seeing is the recurring dream I had in the hospital. Well, I'll be damned. I knew it all along. I just didn't know I knew I'd make it. Nothing to it. You just wander in the desert for forty years, climb the mountain, and there it is all around you. Green, sunny, and fresh. And the view from this side of the mountain is magnificent.

MONTH NINE

Well, life doesn't stay so fresh and breezy. A gentle walk across the field leaves me winded, but I go out there almost every day. And every week I feel a little more energy. The counts continue to rise slowly. I see Offit less frequently. He has stopped the erythropoietin, and the red count has not dropped. No transfusion in almost three months. Which is not to say the counts are normal, but for me, they're better. I work around the house, shop, cook, and do laundry, something to earn my keep.

One day recently in the supermarket, as I wheeled my cart through the diaper section, I was brought up short by a young couple comparing prices while their toddler squirmed in the cartseat. When you change thirty or forty a week, a few dimes' difference adds up. We were buying diapers just last spring. Oh, thank goodness we're finished with them.

But something drew me to this family, and I came back to their aisle to stock up on dishwasher detergent for our first-ever dishwasher. Clare couldn't be more than a year, year and a half, older than this couple's kid, and they were still young enough to have more kids after this one. Suddenly I felt entirely cut off from these people and from the younger half of life. The radiation treatments made me sterile. I will have no more children. Whether I want them or not is not the point. I cannot sire them. I am on the far side of a biological divide. Women facing menopause must feel this separation. This is what it's like for a guy.

Jean and I were given the choice to bank sperm before the transplant. Even before I got sick, we were convinced that two kids were enough for us. No need to bank sperm, "Unless you have some other lady who wants the stuff," she said. No other lady. How, facing all the unknowns of transplant, could we also have decided that I should bank sperm? Would it have meant some very positive thinking—yes, I will survive and want more kids? Something about carrying on into the future? Or would it have meant something entirely morbid—another baby with my genes would be some consolation for Jean if I didn't make it? Or just as morbid—having decided on two kids, what if one of them should fall ill? An extra in the bank? In a two-minute conversation we had agreed: this sperm banking was for younger folk.

But now, here I was in the supermarket, struck dumb and stock still by the realization that this couple was on one side of life's climb, and I was on the other. Biologically, my job was finished. I am not right now dying of cancer, but I am irrelevant to bringing future generations into the world.

My stupor didn't last long. I still have two of the next generation's kids to feed. They are already in this world, and need me to stay in it with them.

MONTH TEN

The red count has reached a decent plateau, and the platelets are a little higher each time they are counted. Both are below normal but not dangerously so. We're fairly well settled into the house, though the furnishings are still sparse. I ride my bike around the country roads and have gone swimming in the college pool, first time in over a year.

I still see Bob Abramson, the acupuncturist, for kind of maintenance treatments. He arranged for me to have a consultation with his mentor and teacher, Leonard Worsley, in New York from London for a conference. "I can't offer this to all my patients."

"But you think I need it?"

"I think you, especially, could benefit from it."

"Then let's do it."

After Worsley's examination, he recommended a treatment plan, which Bob will carry out over the next month or so. The consultation took place in a holistic clinic in Chelsea. I had to rush from a late train to make my appointment. Bob let me into the loft and showed me to a treatment room. I took off my clothes, lay on the paper-covered table, and Bob took my pulses. Then in came an entourage of local practitioners headed by the famous man himself. He asked me a few questions about the diagnosis, the various treatments—especially the transplant—and my family history. "I want to know how you feel about this illness," he asked.

I didn't quite know how to answer. This is a very long and involved question. Judy and I have been talking about it for a year and a half. What can I say in a sentence? He made his question clearer. "What I need to know is how you feel about fighting it. Do you have the spirit?" No one had put the question quite like this before. Not that the question wasn't there, just that I always felt that my presence in whomever's office showed already that I wanted or intended to fight the disease. So many things went quickly through my mind that I became tongue tied. I thought of my mother and the sensation of inevitability that struck me a few days after my diagnosis. I thought of Elizabeth: "You're beating this sucker." Of Gail: "I can't believe he watched his whole bronchoscopy on TV." I thought of the day Richard Collens sent me to the hospital and I cried in the street because Clare might grow up never knowing her daddy. I thought of Jean's quiet, "We'll deal." Of my cousin Judy's, "This plain sucks." Of Judy Nenner's heavy sigh and tears as our story first unfolded to her. Of my answer when Nathan asked if I could die from this cancer: "I have no intention of dying from this." The assembled acupuncturists must have thought me addled that I didn't have a ready answer. Finally, I came out with, "It never occurred to me not to fight it."

"Good," said Worsley beaming, and went on with the next phase of the exam, feeling the pulses. Everybody got a chance. So many warm faces. I've been poked and prodded and felt up by so many doctors and nurses, this group's routine was pretty gentle in comparison. It's not often you get to hold hands with two doctors at once.

"You all have such smooth hands," I said.

"It's pretty cushy work we do," Bob said, and we all laughed.

Worsley took the pulses quickly and passed the back of his hand over my bare chest, testing the body temperature. He pronounced me warm. He had the rest of the crew pass their hands over my chest as he had. I explained that I had rushed to get here in time. They nodded, but clearly I hadn't explained anything.

"Now we will retire and confer," Worsley said. "You relax and enjoy the view." The one window looked out on an air shaft.

I waited. In this, Eastern and Western medicine are identical.

Bob came back. "The others aren't here?"

"Apparently."

"They must be with the other patient." Bob left.

I waited. I wasn't so warm anymore, lying nearly naked on a Chinese table in Chelsea in autumn.

Worsley came in. "Where are the others?"

"That's what Bob wanted to know. I've been relaxing since you left me. Great view."

"The other patient is a model. You know. They must be examining her very closely." The crowd reappeared and gathered around the table. Worsley took up my wrist again, but I wanted to know the results of their conference. "What are you going to do?"

He lowered my wrist, rocked back on his heels, and took a deep breath expanding his white shirt front like a bird about to sing. "First, we are going to treat you. Then, we shall read your pulses again to see how you have responded. If you respond, we shall keep you. If you don't . . . did you see that ash bin on your way in here? That is where we toss you." The crew chuckled.

I sat up on the table. "Oh no," I said, "I've already been to the ash bin."

YEAR FIVE

I am still here. Still breathing, still talking, still tickled to be alive. But no matter what else I say, no matter how glad I am to be in decent health for a guy approaching fifty who survived a bone marrow transplant, who dove down and floated up gasping for breath and is now breathing easily, let me tell you it is not over. It is never over. I am a marked man. I live with one eye over my shoulder and an ear to the ground. No more nasty surprises. Please.

I am reluctant to even breathe the "C" word (not cancer, I can say that one easily enough, but the c-re word) for fear that I will jinx my life and anger the gods. Who are we to think we can beat back the fates with medicine, with our guts emptying from both ends, with fevers, rashes, coughs, infections, lord knows what all, as if enough suffering brings release?

One day shortly before my door was opened, a friend sat at the foot of my bed and joked about the clean gowns and the dirty floor. Then Jane paused for a moment and said, "You are my hero." I was touched but said nothing. I don't think that we who have been through this are heros, and neither are the doctors, nurses, and caregivers saints. We are people hungry for life. Is fifty a full life? Not for me it ain't. Maybe this is what Jane, with her own health problems, meant by hero.

And my transplant was not at all so dangerous as one done with donor marrow. When I think of the additional risks and complications of allogeneic transplant, I am in awe of the courage this takes. Maybe the "allos"—Lini's short hand—are heros. Having had the rotten luck to come down with this disease, I certainly thank my good luck that no lymphoma was detected in the marrow, making me a candidate for autologous transplant.

On my way into transplant, my therapist, Judy, and I talked about death. I'll tell you what I remember saying without vouching for any truth in it. I said, "Death doesn't frighten me. Death is nothing. Dying—I picture a long painful suffocation—scares the shit out of me." Saying this, and knowing that the disease could kill me—so could the procedure, although the chance with autologous transplant was acceptably remote—made me think for a while I could taste death. Perhaps this taste is what Jane meant by heroic: not that we don't all sometimes taste it, but that the transplant patient chooses to. When I sat in the Farber outpatient clinic next to the guys in wheel chairs who had come out the same time I had, and I wondered how they could have been laid so much lower than I and whether I should have been given even stronger medicine, I knew that I had not tasted death—not really, not deeply—or had masked the taste. In the hospital, I had that dream of sunny, leafy, cool comfort, and months later, there I was awake and alive in it. In some deep place I never really doubted that I would come through. Was this faith or knowledge? I had no moment of revelation, no vision of or bargain with god. If there was a touch of the spiritual in this not doubting, it was in my sense of the ordeal as a test: of will, of fiber, of that gnarly knot at the center of the center that hurts and fears and longs and dances and tries to pronounce the unnameable and keeps on breathing.

In optimistic moments, we think we've banked up enough health or suffering or goodness to see us through. Experience and the memory of courage may be stored, but each new crisis has its own demands and chances for disaster. People say to me: You've been through enough, don't "they" know to leave you alone. By "they" they must mean something like the fates. There are no guarantees. Hooray for bone marrow transplantation. I lived to tell the tale. I have dashed across the intersection and the bus has just missed hitting me. Now don't rush, there'll always be another.

But why so wary? you ask. Five years later, how come you won't talk of cure? (You said the "C" word, not me.)

When I first met Dr. Neil Spector at Dana-Farber, a year before transplant, he said, "With you we will probably never talk about cure. We will talk in terms of long-term, disease-free survival." This disease is considered incurable and, even when they have been able to produce long-term remissions with conventional therapies, the disease comes back. So I was warned. Going into transplant, long-term remission sure sounded better than cycles of treatment and partial remission. But if the disease were to be lurking somewhere, my being out of transplant a long time puts me closer to relapse, not further away from the disease. Now you aren't supposed to think like this. Think positive, they tell me. Think, It's gone.

I look at it this way: the wariness keeps the disease at bay. I am not getting caught again. I feel comfort in this wariness, this suspicion. It is work I can still do. People look at me and say, "Oh, you are all better now though, right?" If this is meant to reassure me, it doesn't, though I guess it does reassure them. It is—and I don't for a moment knock this, I live it every day—magnificent to look at a body who's made it through. But for me, late at night or when I've been ill, the wary guard is important. It keeps me company, it keeps me humble, it keeps me actively fighting cancer.

OK, I do feel healthy, and today, this moment is what matters. But my wariness also has some basis in medicine. The chest X-ray has still not cleared. There is less gunk in the lungs but not none. "Extensive scarring" is what the radiologists' reports read. Dr.

Stover, who seems to look at the pictures more carefully than anyone, still saw shrinkage of scar tissue a year after the more cautious radiologists saw "stable scarring." This stuff may or may not be disease. I'm told it may never go away even if it isn't disease. But that it hasn't grown in years is a very good sign. The only way to tell what it is exactly is to surgically remove tissue and look at it under a microscope. But since no one suggests additional treatments now, what would be the point of another thoracoscopy? Must I know? As long as I have no new symptoms, and the disease is at least silent in its corner, and this wariness seems to help keep me healthy, why bother? Some people just have to know. Me, I can take this.

There is one other suspicious sign. There is still cold agglutinin in the blood. Lymphoma can make this antibody and may or may not have in my case. Mycoplasma also makes it, and I had that too. Some doctors think the antibody might linger from the pneumonia, but people with mycoplasma aren't usually followed for years afterward, so who would know? Dr. Offit has wondered if the cold agglutinin could to be the by-product of some other process, one that may have predated my known troubles. Whatever the cause, the titre, like the scar tissue, seems to be stable. And if it comes from residual disease, the level is very low, and/or my body has found a way to keep it under control. Either way it is not causing undue difficulty; I don't even have trouble breathing in cold weather. Since we've moved, I've taken up cross-country skiing. I'm no speed demon, but for a guy with limited lung capacity and an antibody that makes blood lumpy in the cold, I'm doing just fine.

And just in case I might give up my wariness, my years since transplant have not been free of health problems, just free of demonstrated cancer. The transplant has left me more, not less, vulnerable.

At about a year out, I was house-bound for two months with sinus and lung infections. This was a toughy. To be back in bed, feverish and coughing, after just beginning to feel better, was very depressing. More depressing than the struggles of recovering from transplant because it seemed now like backsliding. Have I used the word depressing before? At the time it seemed as if I would never get better. Of course relapse would be more depressing. Locally I had been told, "Yup, ya got the flu like everybody else." I called Gail Schattner at Memorial. She took care of me over the telephone for as long as she could, and when she needed to lay a cool hand on my shoulder, said, "Mr. Seder, it's no surprise your doctor up there doesn't have experience with patients post-transplant. You have to come see us." She was able to diagnose hemophilus influenza, which, unlike viral, is treatable with antibiotics.

I had a brush with Lyme disease. This had nothing to do with transplant, but the enormous fatigue I felt was so familiar from transplant days, it took a pain in the jaw to convince me that this was something different. For this disease, I figured a doctor practicing in the wilds of tic country would be more experienced than an oncologist on the East Side of Manhattan. The Lyme was not advanced and the antibiotic dealt with it. Stupidly I had tricked myself: there is only so much bad business to go around in the world and I have had my share. Out loud I would never have said the transplant somehow made me immune to tic bites, but in the back of my mind I had decided that I was done with disease.

I had laser surgery to repair a hole in the retina, probably caused by aging vitreous in my very-nearsighted eyes. A wash of black specks floating in the eyes showed up only a few months out of transplant. One ophthalmologist said this was caused by slight bleeding and complicated by a still low platelet count. The blood, he said, would take a few months to reabsorb. It hasn't yet.

I have cataracts in both eyes from the TBI. Not bad enough to operate yet, but my vision is a little fuzzy. The cataracts do make the strings of specks a little less visible. About twenty percent of transplant patients wind up with cataracts. Looking at the numbers, this makes immune from other, nastier aftereffects, right? I'm tricking myself again.

I had an absolutely awful bout of the shingles. For a year post-transplant I took acyclovir to prevent herpes infection. A year and a half later—bang, the shingles. Even surgery wasn't so painful as the shingles attacks. The lesions appeared on my left shoulder, up the side of the neck and onto my scalp. When the attacks came, it felt as if a newly fired pot had been taken directly from the kiln and placed on my shoulder. The worst attacks felt as if the hot clay had then melted into the skin.

I had appendicitis. Is this related? My new local doctor has read of a few cases of people post-transplant having trouble with appendicitis. Anybody can get it, but I suppose people post-transplant have trouble with anything. With me the diagnosis was complicated because the doctors expect a very high white count with appendicitis. My white count was still in the "normal" range, but for me high. The surgeon was not terribly impressed until he talked to Dr. Offit. The operation revealed a "bad" appendix and peritonitis.

I spend more time now in dentists' offices—mine and the kids'—than I do in doctors' offices. I still see Bob Abramson every couple of months, and he's a constant source of support and second opinions. After the consult with Worsely, Bob finished his treatment recommendations and afterward continued on his own. Has acupuncture kept me healthy? It hasn't hurt. And when I am ill Bob can usually detect some imbalance and treat it. I don't pretend to understand what he does. I know the mindful attention is helpful. I know that continuing to see him is like my watchfulness, some work I can still do. But I do not want to turn my life into a research project. Should I give up acupuncture to see if I have a relapse?

Just in case I might think maybe I'm in the clear, a clucking tongue warns me off. I enjoy my healthy days when they come. And they are most days now. I no longer design lighting. I teach at my wife's college, a big change, and I am happy with it.

Living through the transplant, I had to keep an eye on the future. If I didn't look through the mess I was living in toward something a bit tidier, what would have been the point? Now that the future is here. I made it. This is the point where the pundits of positive thinking would have me tell you: "Live in the moment. Live for today, who knows what tomorrow will bring?" But it doesn't work quite that way. The disease and treatment shook me profoundly. I remember the moment in the lounge just after my door was opened: I felt I had climbed a great height, and the view from the top was magnificent. As appealing as it might be to dwell at that height, I have come down to ordinary life, and in life we are always looking ahead and looking back, up and down, everywhere but right where we are. I'm caught looking at my feet when there's a gorgeous sunset to see. Look up, dummy. And I do glimpse the sunset just before I focus on the strings of tiny dots floating in my eyes.

Or I sit typing away in a little room while my daughter calls sweetly from the yard. Like any little girl's, her call won't stay sweet long if I don't answer it. She wants to show me something she's made on the lawn. I save your file and go out and look at the

"Indian village" she's built out of sticks. She reminds me that next fall after I cut back the hydrangea stalks, I shouldn't throw them away—like I did last year—because they'll be great for her village. She smiles up at me, and I'm caught between wondering how I'll ever remember her sticks in eight months and wondering if I'll be alive then. Old habit. She goes back to her construction work, but I know I missed something in her eyes while I stood wondering.

I go back to my typing. I do get busy with it. I worry about death and taxes like everybody else. If I don't live in the moment, appreciating every breath, I do live with greater awareness of how close to the moment I am not living. It's right there at my shoulder, and I can be stopped at almost any hour of the day or night and draw an appreciative breath. Something has to stop me though, and lately those somethings have been crowded by other thoughts of teaching and the family. Before transplant, I wasn't so willing to stop or be so appreciative. I cannot but say that my life, what's left of it, is better for this new way of breathing, even with damaged lungs.

Is that sentence wary enough? No more nasty surprises. I wish. I pretend my wariness will somehow protect me from the shock if I should relapse. But you'll see; if it comes I'll be devastated. There is no thorough preparation for cancer or for transplant. There is only time.

The day after my door was opened, I was walking the floor and met the nurse who had given me the first dose of chemo and whom I hadn't seen since. She asked how everything had gone, and I told her the very quick version of what I have told you.

"Oh, you sailed through it," She said.

If you can call getting caught out at sea in a hurricane, sailing.

Afterward

To The Marrow is pieced together from my notes and journals and earlier attempts at a narrative. It is the journal that I would have kept if I could have written more than a few words a day during the transplant.

Anatole Broyard said, “Illness is primarily a drama, and it should be possible to enjoy it as well as to suffer it.” At some times in our lives, we all face serious illness: in ourselves, in our families, or in our work as caregivers. The story of illness is, for many of us, one that insists on its telling. What I have learned through this work is that if one follows it with some attention and diligence, something of—perhaps unexpected—value will come. For those who have wanted to write about their own or another’s illness, the work may not be curative, but it may go some way toward making meaning of tough times.

Robert Seder, January, 2000

In 2001, Bob was diagnosed with myelodysplastic syndrome, which is a kind of early stage leukemia. In September of that year, he endured the more serious and extremely risky bone marrow transplant with tissue from an unrelated donor. Bob and his donor were permitted to write, but not to know each other‘s name or address.

ROBERT SEDER

Note to the Unknown Donor

You don't know me.
I don't know you.
We share something with only
five others in the known world:

A2402
B35nd
C04apa
1104
> > 02
03af
That's us.

You've agreed to give of your very marrow
so that someone somewhere might hope
and live.
I've agreed to be sicker now
so to fight disease
and live.
I know you to be a generous person,
wonderously so.
Being receiver makes me no less a one,
one for longer if not better.

You do not know I am older than you,
but you do know I'm not old enough to say,
That's all, I've had my share.
No, I'm hungry still.

TO THE MARROW

Giving does not protect you.
When your turn comes,
hope some stranger steps forward as you have.
For now your goodness goes noticed and applauded.

We don't know each other,
but I know you are in good health.
You know I'm not.
I can guess you are bigger than me.
Now you know I'm small.
Do you prefer to walk,
to hear your daughter (if you have one) sing to herself,
to remark on the June morning's sun
hitting a north windowsill where it won't again
until we know each other's names?
So we know something.

You don't know me.
I don't know you.
We are (they tell us)
unrelated.
I don't believe them.
Back far enough
we share a great great grand
someone.
Brothers we aren't,
long lost cousins surely.
Lost to whom?

I know you

cherish life or you would never have offered.
You know me
in my fight for life.
We live on
to enrich
the daughters‘ song.